Vicki Caruana's heart is so transparently revealed in her writing that you can't help but be drawn into this book. In its pages, weary teachers will find the roadmap to rest for their souls. Vicki Caruana offers teachers the gift of her wisdom and experience, wrapped in words and stories that engage the heart.

　　—Jennifer Kennedy Dean
　　　Executive Director of the Praying Life Foundation
　　　Author of *Fueled by Faith: Living Vibrantly in the Power of Prayer,* and *When You Hurt and When He Heals*

There have been teaching times when I've cried. There have been times when I've felt exhausted and burned out. And there have been times when I wanted to quit. For all of those times I wish I'd had Vicki Caruana's *Recess for Teachers,* which reminds teachers where to go for rest, comfort, and assurance—to God. Her insightful study never dismisses our very real hurts and frustrations but instead gently directs us to the Savior, who said He would never leave us nor forsake us. If you're feeling thirsty, you'll find lasting refreshment within these pages.

　　—Janet Holm McHenry, teacher, speaker, and author of nineteen books, including *PrayerWalk, Prayerstreaming,* and *Prayer Friends*

13-digit ISBN: 978-0-8054-3124-7
10-digit ISBN: 0-8054-3124-1

Published by Broadman & Holman Publishers,
Nashville, Tennessee

Dewey Decimal Classification: 242
Subject Headings: TEACHERS \ CHRISTIAN LIFE
DEVOTIONAL LITERATURE

1 2 3 4 5 6 7 8 9 10 09 08 07 06 05

Recess for Teachers

taking time out for your body, mind, & soul

Vicki Caruana

Nashville, Tennessee

— To Dad —
I learned how to rest from you.

Contents

Foreword

THROUGHOUT MY growing up years my teachers were my heroes. I loved the way they enjoyed talking about the subjects they were passionate about, and I liked the affirmation I received for doing my homework with excellence. But the teachers who impacted me in the most powerful way were the ones who verbalized their belief in my potential and took the time to make me feel significant. There was energy in their step and enthusiasm in their demeanor. By observing extraordinary teachers, I realized that by choosing a career in education, I could live out my dream of living for something that had lasting value. Several years later I became a speech, drama, and English teacher.

That was only the beginning. I went on to direct an Alternative Education Program for pregnant teenagers, individualizing subjects so my students could stay in school during the duration of their pregnancies. However, after my first six years of teaching, I discovered a new challenge. In spite of my love for my students and my ardent devotion to being the best possible teacher, I was tired. The fatigue started slowly, but it grew into a weariness that started to steal my enjoyment of leisure activities. My mind was always consumed with the papers that still needed to be corrected and the lesson plans that required creativity and future planning. My former joy at the prospect of helping to develop the potential in the students in my classroom was squashed as my fatigue intensified.

Guilt replaced excitement as I looked ahead to the next weeks and months of the school year. I started obsessing on everything I didn't do in a timely manner and on the expectations the principal, the parents, and even the students placed on me. My smiles were forced while I secretly started to regret my career choice. Time urgency and paperwork demanded by the administration made the creative part of education less fun than it was during my student teaching days. My body screamed for rest, and my mind demanded a break. I even sensed less enthusiasm for the development of my spiritual life, which had always been my highest priority.

How I wish I could have met Vicki Caruana earlier in my career! She is trademarked as America's Teacher, and once you meet her—through her best-selling books, as a gifted speaker on educational issues, or in person—you know why! In *Recess for Teachers* Vicki honestly addresses the challenges of the maxed-out teacher who is weary, burned out, and in need of rest.

This book will make you know you are not alone and that there is a time for everything—but you can't do everything at the *same* time. She skillfully weaves biblical principles into real-life illustrations and helps us learn how to experience renewal of the mind, body, and spirit. One of my favorite parts of this book gives testimonials from teachers who give examples of the ways they have learned to be intentional about taking time to rest.

If you picked this book up because you've been tempted to quit, read on. You'll discover that "recess" is as important for teachers as it is for students—and if you are interested in being a good educator, it's as essential to rest as it is to teach. You'll not only want to buy this book for yourself; you'll want to give copies to every teacher you know!

—CAROL KENT, Educator, Speaker, Author
President, Speak Up Speaker Services
Speak Up with Confidence (NavPress)
Becoming a Woman of Influence (NavPress)

Acknowledgments

A NUMBER OF PEOPLE made this book possible and believed not only in the concept of rest but in the teachers who desperately need it. Gary Terashita, my editor, whose belief in this project and my ability as a writer, eased me through the most difficult year of my life. Without his encouragement this book would not be in your hands. David Shepherd and the rest of the incredible publishing staff at Broadman & Holman Publishers diligently prayed for me while I wrote this book. I know the rest I found was a direct result of those prayers. To the teachers who shared how they find rest and renewal, you've offered real-life ways to find rest. And I thank my mother in heaven from whom I continue to learn and who reminded me not to worry because worry steals rest from us.

Introduction

I BEGAN WRITING THIS BOOK as an expression of love and understanding for educators and their desperate attempts to find rest. I know firsthand what it's like to come to the end of yourself as a teacher, yet you're still expected to pour yourself out from an empty vessel. We seem to look for rest in all the wrong places and from all the wrong people. I wanted to help bridge the widening gap between fatigue and rest.

My readers know I write in a very transparent manner. I tell it like it is, and I don't pretty things up just so they'll look good from the outside. I'm much more concerned with the heart than I am with what the world sees on the outside. I think I delivered on that count in this book.

This book came to me at a perplexing time in my life—a time when I couldn't find rest and was guilty of looking for it in all the wrong places. I was a cracked and bitterly empty vessel that couldn't hold water, let alone hope it would divinely discover that it contained wine! I had gone through a difficult, and at times desperate, season of personal grieving, and I started to believe the only way I could be renewed was for this vessel to be shattered into a million pieces so it would vanish altogether. This was my starting point for writing this book. I'm grateful God didn't leave me there.

He taught me about rest step by step. I did shatter and break apart. He did remake me. I did carry water. As I faithfully carried the waters of everyday life, God turned my offering into the best wine! I was empty. He filled me.

If you find you're empty, cracked, or completely shattered, rejoice! This is exactly where God wants you. He will take what you consider the mundane offerings of your work as a teacher and turn them into something precious. He will reward your diligence with peace and rest. It will pass all understanding. It won't make sense because your life really hasn't changed on the outside. You'll still grade papers, still have more paperwork than any CEO, still worry about your students, still struggle with your relationships with students, parents, colleagues, and administrators—yet somehow be at rest. When you walk in obedience, God will turn the water of your everyday experiences as a teacher into the wine of excellence. You can rest and know He is the One who renewed you from the inside out, and everyone will notice.

This book connects your quest for rest with body, mind, and spirit. At the end of each chapter I offer "Rest Stops" (body rest), "Rest Reminders" (mind rest), and "Journal Prompts" (spirit rest). You can use this book for your own personal meditation, or you can open your fellow teachers to the opportunity for real rest.

Part 1

Come to Me

Chapter One

Weariness

"Come to Me, all of you who are weary and burdened,
and *I will give you rest.* All of you, *take up My yoke* and
learn from Me, because I am gentle and humble in heart,
and *you will find rest* for yourselves. For My yoke is
easy and My burden is light."
MATTHEW 11:28–30
(emphasis added)

I HAVE A FRIEND with a thick Texas accent. When she's tired,
I know it! She says, "I'm tard. Pow'rful tard!" As a teacher, I
could utter that statement every day and still not come close to
communicating to my family and friends how tired I really am.
And, boy, am I "tard."

I'm tired mind, body, and spirit. I'm tired when I wake up
and when I go to bed. I'm tired of finding new ways to do the
same thing. I'm tired that very little of what I do makes a difference. I'm tired of not being able to read my students'
minds, say the magic words for parents, and tap into my super-
powers for my administrators. Somehow when I try to explain
this to others who aren't educators, they look at me with con-
fusion. They don't understand why I'm tired. After all, I don't
dig ditches for a living. I don't work twelve-hour shifts like a
nurse, a fireman, or a police officer. I don't stay at home with

three-month-old triplets, wishing I could grow an extra appendage—or two! So why am I so tired? Since you've chosen to read this book, you must be tired of being tired too!

Teaching fatigue is similar to battle fatigue because it's caused by stress and interferes with a teacher's job performance. By the time teachers experience this kind of fatigue, they're burned out and look for ways to leave teaching altogether. Good teachers give more than 100 percent of themselves to their students. It's not surprising they experience debilitating fatigue. The profession and our children can't afford to lose them. One way to extinguish fatigue is to recognize it in its many forms and then set out intentionally to change your thought life, your physical life, and your spiritual life to reflect your desire for rest and renewal.

Mind

Fatigue of the mind encompasses both what you think about and how you feel. Your thoughts and feelings are constantly bombarded by the expectations of everyone around you—parents, students, colleagues, and your own families. You teeter on the edge of overload and think if you could just get away, you could regroup and recharge your batteries. Unfortunately, once on overload, the answer lies not in recharging but in renewal. You must begin anew. Your mental overload comes in the form of too much information over brief periods of time. The expectation to both retain and then implement the information is sometimes more than you can bear. For someone already overwhelmed this can be particularly torturous. Consider the different arenas in which you battle mind fatigue.

INITIATIVE FATIGUE

Hundreds of teaching and learning strategies bombard teachers every year. How teachers do what they do is under scrutiny like never before. In this age of accountability, teachers are expected to meet the needs of each and every child in their care. Although that expectation is a definite desire of every teacher, it may not always be possible. Professors, educational consultants, and researchers all introduce teachers to new and better ways to teach children with the strong belief that *their* way is the best way.

There is no *one* right way to teach. No magic strategy or method ensures all children will succeed. Inside, teachers know this is true, yet they're tempted to believe a quick fix will get the job done. Teachers want so desperately to meet the needs of their students that they're willing to try whatever it takes to get there. The danger here is the belief that it is a *quick* fix. Learning, *real learning,* is a process and takes time. Students respond to consistency more favorably than to constant experimentation. Just because a teacher learns a new strategy that sounds great doesn't mean she must implement it immediately.

To combat initiative fatigue, first give yourself permission to *not* act on every new idea you learn. Then if you fervently believe that change is in order, select a strategy or method that will meet the needs of most of your students. Give the new strategy or method time to make the promised positive impact. Children learn best within a safe, nonthreatening, and consistent environment. If you change the rules, they may become mistrustful of your methods and become apprehensive learners instead of active ones. Count the cost before implementing something new. Predict possible casualties and obstacles to learning and come up with ways to help students adjust to the new strategy or method. Support them in learning new habits. Then at the end of the year, honestly evaluate whether this new initiative made the impact on your students you hoped it would.

TESTING FATIGUE

Teachers have always been intimately involved in testing. Until recently, testing revolved around teachers' created tests or the tests that came with a prepackaged curriculum. *Did my students learn what I wanted them to learn?* Evaluating student progress is a necessary part of the job. In today's climate of accountability, testing has become, more than ever, the tail that wags the dog. We're all painfully aware of the high stakes testing presents. Not only is a child's future at stake but teachers' jobs as well. School image is irrefutably wrapped up in students' test scores. How you respond to the sometimes illogical and impractical nature of district or state testing will determine both the paths of your students and your own as an educator. However, "I test, therefore, I am" is not what drew you to the classroom.

How then can you balance the expectations of the purse-string holders (administrators, school boards, state and federal legislators, and taxpayers) with the desire to meet your students' needs, as varied as they are? The answer is *selected focus*. Teachers are beginning to do just the bare minimum to get by. Going above and beyond the call of duty seems too high a price. But students deserve your best. Choose the important over the urgent. Look at each day as an opportunity to serve students. Expect quality work from students, and enable and equip them to produce it by teaching them to do their work neatly, completely, and correctly, and they will ultimately do well on testing. It's a natural consequence of good teaching.

Focus not on the testing but on assessing. Do your students know the content and can they communicate their knowledge effectively and efficiently?

IN-SERVICE FATIGUE

How often do you roll your eyes at the prospect of yet another teacher in-service day? If you don't approach those days of workshops with enthusiasm, or at the very least healthy curiosity, you're probably facing them with heavy fatigue.

As someone who conducts workshops for educators, I've experienced my share of teachers sitting with their arms crossed and expressionless faces, who look up only to check the clock and whose primary concern is *Where is the food?* Teachers all know what it feels like to teach children who don't care. Can you imagine what it feels like to teach teachers who don't care? Here are three reasons why teachers have an apathetic outlook toward required in-service.

1. *Time away from the classroom* is probably the most common complaint among educators with regard to attending in-service. They have so little time during the school day or week to plan lessons, evaluate students' work, and assess how well they're doing. Meetings and workshops during planning days or teacher in-service days take away the precious little time teachers have. Even service time before the beginning of the school year is full of meetings for both the school and the district. Although some of the offered workshops include ways to refresh, renew, and rejuvenate teaching, what teachers really need is respect for their time so they can find their own ways to be refreshed, renewed, and rejuvenated.

2. *Lack of relevant choices* is another complaint about in-service workshops. While some districts provide an incredible array of learning opportunities for teachers, others offer the same choices year after year. It's not only a matter of variety but of relevance. Do these choices connect directly to the needs of teachers and their students? Often the workshops revolve

around teaching strategies and learner needs. These give the teacher a quiver full of strategies from which to choose but do nothing to meet his own deeper needs.

Look for workshops that closely align with both your philosophical beliefs as a leader and your emotional and spiritual needs as an educator. Usually you're given an opportunity to fill out an evaluation of the in-service. Be honest if your needs aren't met, but then make relevant suggestions you hope planners will take into account for the future.

3. *Unrealistic expectations* are another aspect of in-service fatigue. You may discover much to your delight that what you learn in a workshop can make a real difference in your teaching and students' learning. But the expectations communicated by the leader or the administrators are so high that only failure looms. Either there is a hard deadline attached or a strong sense that if you don't find a way to implement this particular strategy, all is lost. Urgency replaces planning, and you feel compelled to comply whether you really believe you can accomplish the work or not. Some teachers respond to this urgency by plowing forward with fervency, while others, usually more experienced, deem the idea as *unnecessary* and continue on their familiar and safe path.

Your mind swirls with thoughts that threaten to overwhelm and disable. Your effectiveness as an educator depends on clarity of thought and useful habits of the mind. Perception is everything. If you believe something is irrelevant and your mind avoids spending time on it, you won't *do* anything about it. Since what you believe and what you think are irrevocably linked, you must make a conscious effort to examine what you believe to be true about a particular aspect of teaching and make sure your thoughts connect those beliefs to your actions on behalf of students. I will examine these connections more in depth in chapter 7.

Body

The body-mind connection is the subject of much research and discovery. Fatigue of the mind can lead to fatigue of the body. Some symptoms of depression are lack of energy, sleep problems, and chronic illness—all body related. Physical conditions that plague teachers in ways that debilitate can be classified in the following categories.

CHRONIC FATIGUE SYNDROME (CFS)

One of the fastest growing physical complaints among educators is fatigue. How do you know if your fatigue is more than a temporary weakness? Women in particular suffer from chronic fatigue to the point exhaustion gets in the way of doing their jobs. Consider the symptoms of CFS, and see your doctor if you have the first symptom plus four or more of the following symptoms:

- Fatigue that's medically unexplained, of new onset, lasts at least six months, is not the result of ongoing exertion, is not substantially relieved by rest, and causes a substantial reduction in activity levels.
- Substantially impaired memory or concentration.
- Sore throat.
- Tender neck or armpit lymph nodes.
- Muscle pain.
- Headaches of a new type, pattern, or severity.
- Unrefreshing sleep.
- Relapse of symptoms after exercise (also known as post-exertion malaise) that lasts more than twenty-four hours.
- Pain in several joints without swelling or redness.

Physical fatigue that doesn't subside with sleep may indicate other illnesses too. Some of you wait too long before seeking help. You look to Christmas, spring, and summer breaks in hopes of rejuvenation and find yourselves just as tired at the beginning of the new school year as you were at the end of the last. Sleep may not be enough to break the cycle of fatigue. Your doctor may prescribe other measures ranging from vitamin supplements and exercise to prescription drugs and therapy. The goal is to feel more refreshed and rested so you can do the job before you.

VOCAL FATIGUE

Teachers are particularly at risk for developing voice disorders because of certain health problems, habits, or voice use. Teaching requires a great deal of voice use. Vocal fatigue (or impaired vocal stamina) is characterized by a sense of increased effort or strain when talking, accompanied by decreased vocal capabilities (such as volume or quality). It really isn't a matter of whether you're yelling too much in the classroom, but more of a sense that you're using your voice either to challenge an already noisy environment or for prolonged periods of time. Teachers who primarily use the lecture method experience vocal fatigue more often than those who don't. Since talking is one of your greatest tools of communication, you need to take better care of this instrument.

According to the Center for the Voice at the New York Eye and Ear Infirmary, suggestions for teachers talking to groups of people include:

- Drink plenty of water and maintain a healthy lifestyle.
- Use a personal microphone. They aren't very expensive and will help you carry your voice to the back of the classroom.

- Warm up your voice before teaching just as a singer would.
- Balance using your voice with resting your voice. Concentrate more on listening than speaking when you can.
- Quiet the classroom as much as possible before speaking.
- Enlist student participation as much as possible.
- Use nonvocal signals to gain student attention whenever possible.
- Move about the room when speaking. Movement helps keep muscles of the throat and upper body relaxed and helps keep student attention.[1]

Teachers are talkers. But both your vocal cords and your students will thank you if you learn to use your voice more efficiently and effectively.

MUSCLE FATIGUE

Teachers experience muscle fatigue in numerous places. They strain their backs, legs, shoulders, eyes, wrists, and necks because of how they sit, stand, and use the computer. Muscle fatigue can then translate into poor concentration and a general feeling of fatigue. It can definitely get in the way of a job well done.

Back strain results from poor sitting and standing habits. When you sit for long periods of time and don't have a proper chair, you can experience pain and strain in your lower back. Schools are notorious for providing just the bare minimum when it comes to furniture. New schools may do a better job of providing ergonomically correct chairs, but the truth is most teachers use chairs that can actually injure them.

Legs suffer from long periods of standing. Teachers who walk when they talk and circulate the classroom while students are working are more at risk. Although this behavior is effective for keeping students attentive, it can cause muscle fatigue in the legs. Balance your sitting and standing time. Make sure you spend time stretching your legs at the beginning, middle, and end of each school day. Women who wear panty hose should wear the support kind to increase circulation to the legs. Also, be sure to change your position every twenty minutes when possible.

Shoulders, eyes, wrists, and necks all suffer because of increased computer use. The computer has become an integral part of the educator's day. The importance of ergonomically correct and positioned chairs, keyboards, and computer monitors can't be overemphasized. Muscle strains cause headaches, blurred vision, and even dizziness. Carpal tunnel syndrome is a common complaint and can require surgery. Check out the American Federation of Teachers Web site at www.aft.org/psrp/h_s/Pointers/computers.html for health and safety tips at school.

Muscle fatigue in teachers is different from muscle fatigue in athletes. Athletes are encouraged to push through the fatigue in order to ultimately strengthen the muscle. However, teachers' strain and fatigue are because of improper movements and must be corrected in order to prevent injury. Lower back pain, headaches, and blurred vision all contribute to teacher absenteeism. If you find ways to combat this fatigue, you'll have fewer absences.

Spirit

Your spirits, too, can experience fatigue. If you find yourself pulling away from where you worship or friends with whom you worship, that may indicate a sense of weariness in your spirit. If you spend a lot of time being and doing all the right spiritual things, you may experience spiritual burnout. Sometimes God will allow you to come to the end of yourself in all your "doing" so you'll finally *be still* and know Him.

The remedy for spiritual fatigue is knowing when to continue an activity and when to step away. Each issue that follows presents both roads to renewal. To know which way is God's will, you must first *be still*.

PRAYER FATIGUE

At times you feel you're just going through the motions when you pray. Instead of prayer meeting your needs through a dialogue with the Father, it is a rote monologue and you become restless.

WORSHIP FATIGUE

How, where, and when you worship also can become a stumbling block to a fervent pursuit of living your faith. You may find yourself not engaged in the way your church body worships and notice you're merely an observer, sitting in a pew or chair, completely alone among hundreds of people. Worship may seem ritualistic and stale. It's difficult to pinpoint the underlying causes of worship fatigue, but we've all experienced it at one time or another.

The Enemy has a way of demystifying what you hold most sacred. He tries to draw you away from worship with the distractions of unfulfilling rituals, music you don't prefer, or a pastor, minister, or priest whose monotone sermons lull you into a stupor. You back away from the body of believers God has provided and retreat into yourself.

Worship is a very personal pursuit. It's not confined inside a physical church. It can and does occur in your daily life in your job, relationships, and ministries. But when you experience worship fatigue in your chosen congregation, it's time to step back and reassess. Evaluate whether how and where you worship helps you bring glory to God. A change may be in order—a change in you or a change of church. Pulling away may only increase your feeling of isolation, and that in itself doesn't bring glory to God.

STUDY FATIGUE

Have you been to more Bible studies than you can count? Have you found yourself studying the same topics or books over and over? Do you approach the Word of God in a lackadaisical manner? Do you believe you've "been there and done that" when it comes to study of the Holy Scriptures? There's a good chance you're experiencing study fatigue.

If until this point you've depended on the leadership of others to engage you in Bible study, perhaps you haven't taken complete responsibility for your own learning. A leader you don't like or whose style is contrary to your own may color your opinion of the study itself. This instance is one that requires *pushing through* as opposed to pulling away. Just as you hope to engage your students in active learning, so you must pursue it for yourself. Relevance is the key. Choose books or topics of study that correspond with a struggle you're facing or another need. Shake things up by changing formats, groups, or study habits. If your Bible studies usually take place at home by yourself, find a group that meets in the evenings and commit to it. God will redeem the time spent in His Word.

God's Word never returns to Him void, so even if you don't *feel* excited about your study, still you can gain something from it. Try not to depend on emotions to gauge whether your study time is worthwhile. Our hearts are wicked above all things, and even we can't know them. This time of study also will equip you for the ensuing battles you'll face daily in the classroom.

Knowing God's truth and being able to apply it are your strongest weapons against the darkness.

FELLOWSHIP FATIGUE

I admit that when I am hurting or struggling I tend to pull myself away from friends God has placed in my life. The effort it takes to engage in fellowship seems too much. The temptation to pull away from fellowship is strong. When you've spent a lot of time in ministry in your church, you tend to reach a point of burnout, not unlike what you experience as an educator. Everyone needs you, and you begin to believe you're indispensable.

Fellowship is not all about giving. It's also about receiving. Yes, often you are called to minister to others within your church family, but others also are called to minister to you. This is not to say that if you pull away for a time, no one will follow to offer a hand of friendship and support. But you certainly make it more difficult for others to do so if you've secluded yourself. In this case a compromise is called for. You may feel it's important to let go of some activities or ministries so you can heal, regroup, and revive yourself. Try to then also hold onto a few people who understand what your life is like and allow yourself to engage in their lives and them in yours. In this way, they may be just what God designed to help you push through this time of fatigue in your life.

The fatigue you experience as an educator isn't unlike the fatigue all other people feel in their own jobs, families, and life choices. It's real. It does influence what you think about what you do. And it can be debilitating. Your choice of whether to push away or push through the fatigue needs to be something you prayerfully consider and not just react to. When Christ said, "Come to Me, all of you who are weary and burdened, and I will give you rest" (Matt. 11:28), He empathized with your weariness and also promised He was the source of your much-needed rest. Go to Him now in search of God-created rest.

Rest Stops
Eat a balanced diet. You've heard it before—moderation, moderation, moderation!

Rest Reminders
Therefore, whether you eat or drink,
or whatever you do, do everything for God's glory.
1 CORINTHIANS 10:31

When work is a pleasure, life is a joy.
When work is a duty, life is slavery.
MAXIM GORKY

Journal Prompt
Are you experiencing some sort of fatigue? Consider the aforementioned categories and identify your type of physical, mental, or spiritual fatigue. How is this fatigue interfering with your teaching?

Chapter Two

Hats for Sale!

And the peace of God, which surpasses every thought, will
guard your hearts and your minds in Christ Jesus.
PHILIPPIANS 4:7

HOW MANY HATS do you wear? It used to be you could tell
simply by how many hatboxes were stacked in your closet. You
knew you had too many when you couldn't retrieve one without
the rest toppling onto your head and leaving a heap on the floor.
But since wearing hats is no longer the fashion, you now adorn
yourself with the invisible kind. They may be invisible, but they
are no less a necessary part of the wardrobe we call life.

Teachers wear many hats, often at the same time. Think
about the character in the classic children's book *Caps for Sale*
by Esphyr Slobodkina. This cap salesman balances a dozen caps
on his head while he tries to sell them to the townspeople. He
gets very tired and has no money to buy food. So he sits by a tree
and takes a nap. When he awakes, his caps are gone! Up in the
tree where he slept sit monkeys, each wearing one of his caps.
No matter how he tries they won't give them back. Finally, out
of exasperation, he throws his own cap to the ground. The monkeys, great mimickers, follow suit and throw their caps to the
ground. The cap salesman collects his caps and goes back to
town to sell them.

As a teacher, you work hard to balance all your hats—the responsibilities of your profession. But often, at the end of the day, you're weary and don't have anything to show for all the hard work. Sometimes in desperation, teachers walk away, seeking rest. But the escapes you seek aren't always healthy, and your belief that no one can balance the hats the way you do keeps you from finding real rest.

Upon returning you tend to take back all the hats you walked away from, reclaiming your territory. But as you do, you also take back all the things that overwhelmed you in the first place. Is there really a way to balance all your hats, or should you consider paring down your wardrobe?

How do you decide which hats still work with your existing wardrobe and which are so out of style they're never coming back? Which ones make God look good when you look in the mirror? Everything you have is on loan from God in the first place—even your home and your teaching. The desire to take care of and fill the needs of your students is not of your own making. It's your God-given call. Following that call is a light burden compared to balancing dozens of hats.

Becoming overwhelmed, overworked, and at the same time underappreciated is a recipe for disaster. Take control of as much of what is overwhelming as you can. You're the only one who knows how many hats you can wear without falling apart. Others have their own hats issued when they first accepted their teaching positions. Then there are the hats that others have discarded but are still too good to throw out. And there are hats you covet when you spy them in the store window. You take them home and feel so hip and trendy. But as time goes on, these hats don't work with your day-to-day wardrobe and rarely are worn.

Each new responsibility you accept affects how you balance the rest of your responsibilities. Experts, parents, and even your own family and friends all have new ways to improve your quality of life that they'd like you to try. You can't wear every hat offered, but you can choose a new one every once in awhile. The key is balance; when you put on a new hat, take off an old one first. Each new activity, strategy, and even friendship needs to be carefully considered before you integrate it into your already top-heavy routine. Try to balance rest and work. And if you take a nap under a tree, don't worry if monkeys steal your hats. You're probably better off without them anyway!

Things to Remember While Wearing Hats

Your responsibilities as a teacher don't exist in isolation. You also have responsibilities as a family member, friend, member of a larger community, and as a child of God. Some of these responsibilities are unavoidable, while others are basically a matter of will—you make a choice.

MATCH YOUR PRIORITIES AND ACTIONS

What you believe is important and what you value is usually revealed through how you spend your time, money, and talents. What do you value as a teacher? As a parent? As a human being? If you don't always act or make decisions based on your values, this causes both inner and outer strife and can lead to a great deal of unrest.

Teachers who say they believe a nonthreatening learning environment is important, yet find themselves yelling often, experience a great deal of frustration and even disappointment in their own actions. There's nothing wrong with valuing a nonthreatening learning environment, but if you find yourself unable to put your priorities into action, something's wrong. Educators all believe in a certain educational philosophy, but putting that philosophy into practice is another story. Take time to reevaluate your priorities and determine whether you truly subscribe to what you say you believe. Then make sure what you do in your classroom and with kids matches what you believe is really important. You can then let everything else fall away and find peace.

LET GO OF THE CARES OF THIS WORLD

If you let go of cares, you can really care for God's children instead. There are many times you find yourself paying much more attention to the urgent instead of the important. Your daily demands are great, and you're required to do many more things besides actually teach. You get bogged down by paperwork, testing, committee duties, and the expectation to implement new technologies in your classroom. It feels like a tug-of-war, and you're losing ground!

Children around you may be struggling, and you eye them peripherally. You want to give them your time, but there doesn't seem to be enough to go around. Meeting every deadline and filing every piece of paper mean nothing if a student falls through the crack on your watch. You didn't go into teaching for the paperwork; you went into it for the children. As God has put them in your care, you must focus on meeting their needs and setting them up to succeed. As far as paperwork is concerned, remember, "Tomorrow is another day!"

NO ONE IS INDISPENSABLE

Teachers are made to feel they're indispensable. Admittedly, it's not easy to fill the shoes of a good teacher. Every substitute relates to that challenge. Every principal is painfully aware of the hole a good teacher leaves when she's absent or moves to another school.

When I was preparing to go on maternity leave, I was consumed with choosing just the right replacement. I wanted to ensure that the person taking my place would continue my work with students with the same diligence and expertise. I worried that students wouldn't get what they needed and begin to fall behind. That concern may be admirable, but it's not practical nor realistic. Nature abhors a vacuum. A hole will not remain a hole; it will be filled. Just remember, it may not be filled with the same substance or quality you would prefer, but it will be filled. It may not always be the best for your students, but they will adapt.

MEDITATE ON SCRIPTURE

Choose an inspirational Scripture verse and meditate on it daily. I know teachers who post inspirational and motivational quotes all over their classrooms to encourage students. They want their students to begin to think, believe, and then act on those sayings. Surround them with positive thoughts and they will begin to think more positively.

What about you? How do you stay motivated and inspired? God's Word is powerful. It can save and change lives! Look for verses that inspire you and post them nearby—on your desk, your computer screen saver, as part of a perpetual calendar, and in your plan book. Begin and end each school day with a reminder from God's Word of your real source of strength and rest.

GOD IS FAITHFUL EVEN IF PEOPLE LET YOU DOWN

Schools are human institutions. They're filled with people who fail and let you down. They're full of sinners—just like churches. Why then are you surprised when schools don't come through, don't fulfill promises, or forget their responsibilities altogether? To be honest, you have to admit you don't always do everything right either. Even other Christian teachers will let you down. As discouraging as this may be, keep in mind that sometimes God allows even those you trust the most to fail so that you'll remember the One who is truly faithful. God is always faithful, even if everyone else lets you down. This isn't to say you shouldn't expect the best from others, but don't be disillusioned either when they fail.

THANK GOD DAILY FOR THE CALL TO TEACH

The call to teach is a way to serve Him. Teachers are doers, very busy people involved in a variety of activities. You thrive in what others see as chaos. Multitasking is great, but if you mistake all you do as a teacher as separate from what you do as a child of God, you've missed your calling.

Too often we look at work we do at church as God's work and the work we do at school as *our* work. There's no distinction. It is all God's work. Don't feel you have to involve yourself in a variety of ministries at your church in order to fulfill a Christian duty quota. Your calling to teach God's children is ministry. And it can be all-consuming. Leave the guilt of volunteering behind you and walk forward in your call as a teacher.

Ways to Remove Hats

It's one thing to manage all the hats you wear. It's quite another to make a conscious effort to remove some of these hats and actually discard them. Some hats are probably getting in your way not only of rest but of doing a good job as a teacher. Don't wait for someone else to come along and take them from you. Remove them yourself.

LIGHTEN YOUR LOAD

If others can do it, let them. Teachers tend to be territorial. We rely on our expert status so heavily we don't know how to ask for help when we really need it. Some of us wouldn't know what to do with a parent volunteer if we had one every day! Sometimes in the quest for more respect, prestige, and even a new position, we even take on more duties in order to impress.

You may not be able to admit it, but the truth is that you say *yes* in order to please someone else. It's not necessary to grab every opportunity at school to gain the respect of your colleagues or superiors. If your load *feels* too heavy, it probably is. And if your load is too heavy, you won't be able to do your best job. If you've already said yes to too many things, look for others who can bear some of the load instead. This is not a matter of defeat. It's a matter of being a good steward of your time and talents to educate children.

ORGANIZE FOR MAXIMUM EFFICIENCY

An organized space is a peaceful space. Although some claim to operate effortlessly among chaos, most people aren't comfortable in such a space. If you can't find what you need when you need it, stress results. Students aren't the only ones who misplace assignments. Sometimes teachers do too. Beginning teachers are notorious for being disorganized. It's a rude awakening to discover the mounds of papers that cross your desk on any given day. Learning how to manage information more efficiently will relieve your stress and student or parent unrest. If organization is something you struggle with, look at some of your colleagues' classrooms. Find someone who looks as if he's got it together and ask him for suggestions. Everyone will appreciate your job efficiency, and you will finally find some semblance of peace in your surroundings.

PLAN QUIET TIME

Take the few minutes before students arrive as a personal quiet time. Some teachers arrive early before students to read the newspaper. They claim it's the only quiet time they have at school or at home. They're probably right. But instead of the newspaper, read from the Bible or a favorite devotional. Maybe read down your roster and pray briefly for each of your students. This is precious time. It may be your only chance to commit your works to the Lord for the day. Your own spiritual growth and the well-being of the children in your charge deserve this time.

READ FOR PLEASURE

Even though you read for information, make it a point to read for pleasure as well. When was the last time you read a novel? Teachers tend to be readers, but you've spent so many years reading to learn about teaching that you're too tired to read for pleasure. You don't have to be too ambitious. Try to read one chapter or commit to reading fifteen minutes a day. Find a time of day when you won't be interrupted. Reading just before bed might put you to sleep, but if you read for only fifteen minutes it will be a welcome lullaby.

SPEND TIME WITH FAMILY AND FRIENDS

During the evenings and weekends, enjoy time with family and friends before you correct papers or plan lessons. Your life is so busy that family time just falls by the wayside. You spend more time driving your children to activities than engaging in activities *with* them. The pile of history day projects may be sitting on your kitchen table, but family still comes first. Spend time with your family first, then spend time working. It's a matter of negotiation. "I'll play Scrabble with you now, but then I need to grade papers for the hour after that." There will always be papers to grade, but your family will not always be available. Let yourself off the hook—family comes first!

PAMPER YOURSELF

Whether you just melt at the sight of good chocolate or yearn to go hiking in the foothills, it's important to do the things you truly enjoy. If you never spend time doing the things you love, you may become resentful of your job. Who wants to be taught by a frustrated and resentful teacher? Who wants to work next door to one? Stop waiting for someone else to come along and pamper you. You know what you need—give it to yourself!

Wearing too many hats not only looks silly, it's dangerous. If balance is the key, keep in mind that a person can balance only so many hats without them crashing to the ground and taking others down with them. It isn't really whether you're better at balancing than someone else. It's whether you should be wearing all those hats in the first place.

You Know You're Wearing Too Many Hats When . . .

- You find yourself still exhausted even after a great night's sleep.
- Conversely, you may be having trouble sleeping.
- You arrive at school and leave with the bell.
- You become forgetful about the important things.
- You're taking more and more sick days.
- Your patience is threadbare.
- You criticize any new idea presented about how to improve teaching and learning.
- You find yourself drifting or daydreaming during important conferences or meetings.
- Your end-of-the-year countdown begins in October.

Individual symptoms may vary, but keep in mind that you're not the only one experiencing the consequences of your top-heavy life. Your students will feel your frustration, anxiety, and disappointment about your job. Parents will know it when they come to you for help about their child. A healthy, happy classroom begins and ends with the teacher.

Rest Stops
Exercise in moderation. Regular exercise results in deep, restful sleep, increased energy and vitality, enhanced decision-making ability, enhanced feelings of well-being, greater clarity of mind, and reduced anxiety, depression, and tension.[2]

Rest Reminders
Whatever you do, do it enthusiastically,
as something done for the Lord and not for men.
COLOSSIANS 3:23

Journal Prompt
Think about the hats you wear. If you could discard
any, which would go? Remember that what you hold is a
choice. Will you let some of your burdens go?

Chapter Three

There's a Time for Everything—
Just Not All at the Same Time

Better one handful with rest,
than two handfuls with effort and pursuit of the wind.
ECCLESIASTES 4:6

MY THOUGHTS SWIRLED and blew violently through my mind like the winds outside. The trees surrounding our home threatened to release their dead branches onto our roof. I sat in our glass-encased sunroom at midnight unable to see the wind, yet hearing and seeing its results all around me. I wondered if our patio furniture would stay put. In my mind, I checked and rechecked whether every window was closed. I heard our metal mailbox flapping open and closed just outside the front door, reminding me that not everything was secured. Yet it wasn't important enough for me to go outside and fasten it. I sat motionless waiting for the howling to stop, so I could finally go to bed without worry.

Have you heard about those who call themselves storm chasers? Their hope is to get close enough to a violent storm or

tornado to study it and then share with the rest of the world
what they discovered. Although many are scientists determined
to improve weather prediction in order to save lives, they all
admit that the thrill is in the chase. But even if they do uncover
an important meteorological discovery, they are still chasing
after the wind.

King Solomon is probably quoted more than anyone else in
the Old Testament, by believers and nonbelievers alike. His
proverbial wisdom stands the test of time. If we will look at our
lives and teaching careers as seasons, we will be able to keep
everything in perfect perspective. As teachers we attempt to do
everything, on our own, all at the same time. No wonder we're
tired. No wonder we begin to believe that it's all meaningless. As
the hurricane force winds surrounded our home that night, I
reminded myself that all within those walls were merely things,
and in the grand scheme, they were meaningless. Trying to hold
onto them for their own sake was like trying to hold onto the tail
of a tornado. As we find ourselves desperately trying to hold
onto all the winds of change that swirl around us as teachers, we
need to let go and focus instead on the glory of God that
grounds us.

Let's focus on the third chapter of Ecclesiastes for timely
advice and admonition:

> *There is an occasion for everything,*
> *and a time for every activity under heaven:*
> *A time to give birth and a time to die;*
> *a time to plant and a time to uproot. (vv. 1–2)*

School has a particular and recognizable ebb and flow.
There is enthusiasm on the first day. There are quarter, semester, and year endings. At times you begin new projects and
processes or change classrooms, grade levels, and even schools.
When you recognize this ebb and flow, you can ease into each

transition instead of fighting it. Don't let the constantly changing landscape take you by surprise and rob your joy.

A time to kill and a time to heal;

a time to tear down and a time to build. (v. 3)

There are times to scrap everything and move on. Maybe you came up with a project for your students that didn't work out. It may feel humiliating to admit it was poorly designed or executed, but it's better to stop something that isn't working and revise the idea. Sometimes what you do in your classroom can inadvertently hurt students. You may not take the needed time to make sure each child understands a particular concept. This leaves some students behind. In your quest to finish on time, you forget to extend grace to a child whose spirit is wounded or whose understanding is cloudy. You can prevent much disillusionment and disappointment with good planning. Take time to plan. That time will later be redeemed and your outlook refreshed.

A time to weep and a time to laugh;

a time to mourn and a time to dance. (v. 4)

We teachers somehow think we need to keep our personal feelings separate from how we relate to our students. Some of us follow the adage "Never smile before Christmas." Others are afraid of blurring the line between teacher and friend. Fear that our authority will be compromised drives us to remain as stoic as possible. I know plenty of teachers don't bridle their emotions and share them freely with students.

But for those of you who worry about being too human in front of kids, be encouraged that there is a time for even surprising giggles and stray tears. If the class clown is actually funny, go ahead and let yourself laugh once in awhile. If the chicks died in the incubator, share your tears with students. And if your track team wins the state championship, do the happy dance! Your humanness makes you more approachable to students. Allowing yourself to respond true to your emotions is much less stressful as well.

A time to throw stones and a time to gather stones;
a time to embrace and a time to avoid embracing. (v. 5)

Even with all your planning, at times you can allow the student interest to drive the curriculum. If you follow the scope and sequence closely, you miss opportunities to let kids get excited about what they're learning and investigate more fully the subject matter. Some educators believe these detours or rabbit trails are not productive. But every journey benefits from a detour now and then. It adds interest and even drama. Taking time to go more in depth with students is like stopping to enjoy a scenic overlook during a long, tiresome trip; you need a break from the road. The balance comes in knowing when to make a pit stop and when to keep going. Sometimes you must gather everyone together and get back on track so you eventually get where you're going. Stay open to the possibilities and relieve yourself from the belief that all will be lost if you don't keep moving. You'll find yourself breathing more evenly and smiling more often.

A time to search and a time to count as lost;
a time to keep and a time to throw away. (v. 6)

Teachers are always hunting for new and better ways to motivate kids, be more efficient, make their classrooms more enjoyable places to learn, find cheap and even free materials, and make their teaching more exciting for students and themselves. Some are gifted at grant writing. Others are creative with small budgets and few supplies. Still others make their classrooms so cozy no student would ever want to go home.

Another aspect is that teachers are pack rats, not just physically but emotionally. They hold onto outdated ideas, ways of doing things, and materials.

As children change, you must, too, if you hope to reach and teach them. How things worked with your last class may not work with this one. You may also hold onto previous hurts from students, colleagues, administrators, and parents. Those hurts paralyze your ability to meet the needs of students and bring glory to God. You must release these hurts and move on to find real rest.

A time to tear and a time to sew;
a time to be silent and a time to speak. (v. 7)

There is a time to undo what you've done and a time to do again what you've undone. Sometimes that means you must fix something you've done wrong. If you've been angry and taken your anger out on students or mistreated someone in any way, you need to recognize your guilt, grieve over it, and show that you know you've done wrong. The next step is to restore any broken trust or broken relationships. Education is all about relationship. If you can't humble yourself to admit when you're wrong, you won't be the teacher your students need you to be.

There will be times it's necessary to sit in silence and listen, and there will be times you must speak. Learning how to talk so parents will listen and listen so parents will talk is the key to effective communication, and effective communication is the key to a healthy relationship. Relationships can cause a great deal of stress, but if you actively look for ways to improve them, you'll find peace.

A time to love and a time to hate;
a time for war and a time for peace. (v. 8)

With those inside and outside your sphere of influence, there's a time to love, to be friendly, free, and cheerful. These are wonderful times when you believe the giving of yourself is best. But there may come a time you feel betrayed by old friends, and you may need to break off ties. Maybe a teacher of whom you were quite fond does something inexcusable and hurtful to either a child or to another innocent party. If there is unrepentant sin, creating a safe distance is recommended. There also may come a time when what was once done in secret is revealed by the light, and God's judgment drops like a deadly sword.

If you've experienced a time of injustice, either toward yourself or a student, be prepared for a time of war. Fighting for the rights of children is part of your job as teacher. Even during a time of war, you can hope for peace when justice is served and God brings reconciliation. There are times to tremble during the war and rest in the peace that follows. Neither will be everlasting, neither war nor peace. Don't let spiritual warfare take you by surprise. Even during a terrible fight in which God has placed you, He is the one in control, and you can have peace even when no peace is found.

What does the worker gain from his struggles?
I have seen the task that God has given people to keep them
occupied. He has made everything appropriate in its time. He
has also put eternity in their hearts, but man cannot discover
the work God has done from beginning to end. (vv. 9–11)

Labor and toil have been a part of God's plan for humanity since the fall of Adam and Eve. Toil is the ultimate burden. Work is supposed to be hard. There is a purpose behind the hard labor, however. It's a constant reminder that on Earth is not where we find the rest we long for. It sets our hearts on eternity. It sets our sights on the only One who can bring that rest. It's hard for us to see the big picture and how God has woven it all together to prepare us for living with Him in heaven. Yet He has done it!

The frustrations of teaching and dealing with students are a part of the prep work. We may be able to find small pockets of rest here and there, but the only refreshing rest comes when we leave the state testing, difficult parents, minuscule budgets, unreliable colleagues, misplaced administrators, and under-performing students at His feet and set our eyes on our future home. So what do we gain from all this trouble and toil? We finally see things as God does.

> *I know that there is nothing better for them than to rejoice and enjoy the good life. It is also the gift of God whenever anyone eats, drinks, and enjoys all his efforts. (vv. 12–13)*

We teachers aren't born teachers, nor do we ourselves choose to be teachers. Our job is to do good. I believe that the majority of us who go into teaching do so because we love kids and desire to make a positive difference; we want to do good! There is pleasure in doing good. School years are short, and students come and go quickly. We really have little time in which we can do good, so we must do whatever we can to stay focused on that task and redeem the time. As each new school day dawns, we can take advantage of the pleasure God gave us for doing good. He created that pleasure for our sakes. We can pur-posely enjoy and rejoice in the good of our labor. It's God's gift to us. When a child smiles or finally grasps a long-studied con-cept or when a parent says you made the difference that year, enjoy God in the good. Give Him the thanks and serve Him with a joyful heart. Even when the earthly rewards seem few and far between, any good that we do and pleasure we experience are from God's abundance.

> *I know that all God does will last forever;*
> *there is no adding to it or taking from it. God works*
> *so that people will be in awe of Him. (v. 14)*

God's design on your life is perfect. It may not look perfect, but if you could see it laid out in front of you, there would be nothing you would be able to add or take away. Nothing is wasted. Even if you find yourself on the verge of quitting and leaving teaching behind, your time was not wasted. When you question why you went into teaching in the first place, the answer comes in God's will. You were and continue to be right where He designed you to be. Why must you experience the weariness and restlessness that accompany your call? So you might see His perfect will and desire to bring your will to His.

At this point you may have tried anything and everything to find rest and renewal as a teacher. You may be struggling to find a reason to stay. You may feel beaten and brokenhearted. You may feel you're in the middle of a whirlwind being tossed from one end of the spectrum to the other. You want to have everything under control, and you want to make sure everything that could be done was done. If Ecclesiastes can teach you anything, it's that your toil is not for your own sake; it's so you can do good to those in your charge. Children are in your charge. They deserve your best. The source of your rest is not found in days off, summer breaks, or snow days. It's a gift from the heavenly Father who from His abundance gives you a taste of what toil and trouble are preparing you for—the loving rest of heaven.

Rest Stops
Practice gentle physical and breathing exercises to calm your body and mind.

Rest Reminders
The LORD will always lead you,
satisfy you in a parched land,
and strengthen your bones.

You will be like a watered garden
and like a spring whose waters never run dry.
ISAIAH 58:11

All outside is lone field, moon and such peace,
Flowing in, filling up, as with a sea,
Where upon comes Someone, walks fast on the white,
Jesus Christ's self . . .
To meet me and *calm all things back again.*
ROBERT BROWNING
(emphasis added)

Journal Prompt
What new perspective have you gained from this
brief study of Ecclesiastes? Are any pursuits you claim
as a teacher in reality chasing the wind?

Chapter Four

Following Directions

The fear of the LORD is the beginning of wisdom;
all who follow His instructions have good insight.
His praise endures forever.
PSALM 111:10

EVERY GREAT ADVENTURE results from following people who are on a quest. Whether it's a classic novel turned into a motion picture, a role-playing game, or this Christian life, people of character journey into the unknown with a lofty purpose. They must gather supplies and equipment, devise a plan of action, and overcome obstacles and regroup when necessary. They must persevere until the very end. If specific directions are given, they must follow them or risk losing the very thing they pursue. And they continue to learn more about themselves every step of the way.

Early in my education to become a teacher, I discovered there was much to learn. Each class I took filled my head with instruction about how to teach this or how to teach that. It was and continues to be the greatest "step" program I've ever experienced. It was good preparation for when I had my own classroom.

Success results from following those steps, so you begin to indoctrinate your students to follow directions as well. You break every concept, every task, into manageable steps and require students to show their work so you know whether they've followed the steps. And when a child fails to master a concept, you look first to see if he had trouble with a particular stage. From setting up classroom rules to conducting a semester project, following directions brings peace and success. It can mean the difference between chaos and tranquility.

As you consider why you struggle to find rest as a teacher, look at the different steps and see where you've made careless errors or didn't grasp the concept at all. First, you must know your objective. Then you can gather materials before setting in motion the procedure to find rest. If you haven't mastered the concept, it's time to evaluate skills and review where necessary. This may sound didactic for such an abstract concept as rest, but teachers are great at following directions and appreciate the clarity this approach provides.

The Objective

Sometimes it's hard to pinpoint what you really need. Do you need more sleep? Maybe you want to eliminate behavior problems in your classroom. Maybe you need to find more time for your family. Have you taken on too many responsibilities and aren't doing any of them well? Are you having difficulty finding time for God? Take time to identify what hinders you from finding rest and renewal. There may be a variety of obstacles, but if you had to choose the one hindering you the most, what would it be?

Emotions can get in the way of your quest for rest. One way to approach the problem objectively is to define it succinctly after you've identified it. For example, use this phrase: "In what ways might I . . . ?" The following questions may help you:

- In what ways might I carve out quiet time during the school day?
- In what ways might I get home earlier to my family each night?
- In what ways might I regain a sense of peace with students in my classroom?
- In what ways might I keep in better contact with parents?
- In what ways might I build more positive relationships with colleagues?

Put into words your goals for rest using this format. You may find more than one thing is bothering you. Can you identify each as being a mind, body, or spirit need or desire? If you have more than one, keep in mind it's more effective to work on one at a time. Prioritize your goals.

The Materials

No lesson is well prepared without first determining and then gathering the necessary materials. How often have you had a great lesson plan only to discover at the last minute you couldn't get your hands on the materials you needed? Poor planning is the culprit, and students lose out.

As you plan for much-needed rest and renewal, you must take the time to gather what you'll need to make rest a reality. There's nothing more frustrating than knowing what you want but not having what you need to get it. Rest doesn't just happen. Careful planning of your days and tasks will open up welcomed pockets of renewal.

Think of the objective you've stated above. What will you need in order to accomplish it? Let's consider materials necessary for the following objectives:

In what ways might I carve out quiet time during the school day?

Materials: an inclusive list of tasks for the day, schedule of required meetings, getting to school a few minutes earlier than usual, Bible, devotional, prayer journal or other inspirational/meditational material, and the willingness to make whatever changes are necessary to achieve this goal.

In what ways might I keep in better contact with parents?

Materials: addresses and phone numbers of parents, a way to monitor and organize parent e-mails or phone calls, a monthly newsletter e-mailed from your classroom, the desire to build better relationships with parents.

As you can see, the materials necessary for your objectives will be physical, emotional, and sometimes spiritual in nature. Sometimes you may believe you have all your ducks in a row, yet leave out the most crucial ingredient—the desire or willingness to change.

The Procedure

Normally I wouldn't quote the Three Stooges, but in their movie *Gents without Cents,* Moe is under posthypnotic suggestion. When Curly says "Niagara Falls," Moe turns on him and says, "Slowly I turn, step by step, inch by inch." Moe pursues a calculated course of action. He does it slowly and intentionally.

You shouldn't need posthypnotic suggestion to help you achieve your goal of rest. Yet you can identify step by step what you need to do. If you've been living with restlessness for a long time, change may come slowly. The bigger the ship, the longer it takes to turn it!

Consider the objective you identified at the beginning of this chapter. Now that you've gathered your materials, what are the steps to accomplishing this goal? Let's continue with the example to illustrate the process.

In what ways might I keep in better contact with parents?

Materials needed: addresses and phone numbers of parents, a way to monitor and organize parent e-mails or phone calls, a monthly newsletter e-mailed from your classroom, the desire to build better relationships with parents.

Step 1: Look at the calendar and choose one day per week to call parents.

Step 2: Check e-mail daily before school starts.

Step 3: Answer e-mail before leaving for the day.

Step 4: Send out a brief classroom newsletter once a month to keep parents updated about what's going on in your classroom.

Step 5: Call parents to tell them something positive about their child. Commit to calling each parent by the end of a quarter.

Step 6: Create a folder in your computer to keep parent messages by student name.

Step 7: Remember, you're building relationships that can only benefit students.

There is no time limit on these steps. If you've never been this intentional about creating a new habit or achieving a goal or desire, you may be tempted to rush things. Real change takes time. Take one step at a time.

Assessment

Sometimes you think you're doing what you're supposed to do and are blinded to your deficiencies. In order to take an honest inventory about how well you are achieving your desired goal, you may have to enlist the help of someone you trust.

One particularly stressful year, I felt more overwhelmed than usual. It disabled me to the point that even my family relationships were beginning to break down. I made a list of all my tasks to see if I was doing too much. At first glance it looked manageable. Then I gave the list to my husband to get his take. He laughed out loud and said, "You missed a couple of things, hon." I gave him permission to add to what I believed was an exhaustive list, and he added more than twenty items! I was shocked and certain he was making it up. He wasn't. He just added the daily things I took for granted and did without thinking—laundry, preparing meals, grading papers, taking our children to sporting events. I crumbled into a defeated heap. Why couldn't I see clearly where I'd gone wrong?

At times, even after your best efforts, you still fail. In the above example—*In what ways might I keep in better contact with parents?*—I've failed, even after following my plan of action. The danger comes when you can't admit failure and become defensive instead. I've had parents emotionally bruised when I believed I had done everything I was "required" to do in order to maintain contact. The problem was, doing what was required was not enough.

To truly find peace and rest as a teacher, first honestly evaluate whether you're really doing what is *right,* not just what is required. Self-assessment is a necessary component of finding rest. Ask yourself why you do what you do—before someone else does.

Show Your Work

I remember the first time a principal observed me in action before my annual evaluation. I was petrified. Not only because I had no idea what to expect, but because I felt on display. My teaching style, my behavior management choices, and my expertise were all out in the open for anyone to see and criticize. I was blessed with a principal whose criticism fueled my drive to become the best teacher I could and did not destroy my newfound confidence. I admit my first response to his evaluation was one of defensiveness, but soon afterward I examined the validity of his suggestions. Not only did he speak truth, but the evidence documented on the evaluation was accurate. I had to admit I still had a lot to learn.

You require students to show their work not so you can torture them or mock their attempts but to be able to pinpoint careless errors or holes in learning. The goal is to find the way to improve. You, too, must be willing to show your work. Your self-protective nature sometimes prevents teaching with transparency. Many teach with complete confidence, yet even they wouldn't want their works on display and under scrutiny.

It's time to evaluate whether how you're doing what you're doing is working toward your goal. Look at your stated goal and determine if anything needs tweaking. In the example *In what ways might I keep in better contact with parents?* you might find you still receive more e-mails from parents than you can answer or a monthly newsletter is not feasible with your available time. When something's not working, you have two choices. Either discard it and come up with another solution or persevere, hoping that in time it will work. Some solutions take time to work. You must be patient enough to watch them come to fruition.

Reteach

Good teachers can recognize a gap in learning. Great teachers do what it takes to fill that gap. It's one thing to identify a problem, but it's quite another to take steps to solve it. Math is one of the more obvious subjects in which it's imperative there are no learning gaps. Each concept builds on the last, and one missing skill or lack of understanding can eventually cause cascading failure. Watching a child try to move forward when he doesn't understand a fundamental concept is like watching him slowly drown. Teachers must decide quickly if they're going to stop what they're doing, leave the safety of the ocean liner they're piloting, and rush headfirst into the water to save him.

There will be things you'll have to relearn for yourself if you're going to do what it takes to make a change in your life. If you can pinpoint what went wrong in your plan of action to achieve your goal, you can work on that one element. Maybe you're not as organized as you could be and maintaining the list of parent contact information threw you for a loop. Find out how to improve your organizational skills. Is there a teacher whose prowess at keeping an orderly work area you admire? Humble yourself and ask her how she does it. Find out where you need improvement and then just do it.

Usually I know what's best for me and what steps I must take to achieve desired rest. Unfortunately, I don't always do what I know I must. I know I should walk more. Walking helps me to sleep better. When I sleep better, I feel renewed and refreshed and I handle daily stresses better. Getting myself to actually go for a walk is the challenge. Figuratively and literally, I need to put one foot in front of the other!

Reevaluate

After you reteach and children relearn, it's time to reevaluate their progress. This is the process of continual improvement. You can't assume that just because you went over the material again the student actually learned it. Testing and retesting skills are necessary to determine mastery. The same is true as you consider the goals you've set for yourself.

One way to determine whether you've met the goal of *keeping in better contact with parents* is to solicit feedback from parents themselves. Your perception of how you're doing may be different from someone else's. Self-evaluation is one thing; peer evaluation is quite another.

For your personal goal of finding rest and renewal, your own assessment of whether you've achieved it is important. However, those close to you may also be able to tell you whether they notice a renewed sense of peace in you. My husband knows when I'm more stressed than I can handle. If I ask him to give me honest feedback, he will. Am I willing to hear his analysis of my current state of being? I must be if I want to finally find the peace I desperately need.

There is more than one way to do almost everything. The only thing carved in stone is the way to heaven. Even then you must follow directions. Believe in the Lord Jesus Christ and you will have eternal life. What is the goal? *In what way might I have eternal life?* What are the materials necessary? *Faith in Christ alone.* What is the step-by-step procedure? *Believe in the Lord Jesus Christ.* Faith is continually tested. It's perfected day by day. The only difference here is there will be no opportunity to reteach if you get it wrong!

Seize the opportunity now to find your way to your desired goal of rest and renewal. It won't come on its own. It must be pursued. God said to enter into His rest (Heb. 4:10–11). He said, "Remain in Me, and I in you" (John 15:4). *You* must take the first steps toward rest. Step by step and inch by inch.

Rest Stops
Cultivate healthy sleep habits. Stop eating sugar at night!

Rest Reminders
Rest in God alone, my soul,
for my hope comes from Him.
PSALM 62:5

It is right to be contented with what we have,
but never with what we are.
SIR JAMES MACKINTOSH

Journal Prompt
Spend time identifying your problems, determining
your materials, and setting into motion your plan for
rest. Commit these ways to the Lord and move forward
step by step. After all, you're on a quest for rest!

Part 2

Take My Yoke

Chapter Five

His Yoke Versus Our Yoke

Christ has liberated us into freedom. Therefore stand firm
and don't submit again to a yoke of slavery.
GALATIANS 5:1

HAVING RAISED HIS CALF from birth, a boy no older than
my own fourteen-year-old son harnessed his pride and joy with
an obviously older and stronger ox in a wooden yoke. The difference in size was almost comical. It was certainly an uneven
pairing. But this was the only way the young ox could learn how
to steadily walk the rocky path. The boy watched as the two tra-
versed the barren soil. The younger stumbled more than once
and at times felt his neck pulled back to center when he took his
eyes off the path. The older ox carried the brunt of the load and
kept the newly plowed furrow straight. In time, the young ox
would learn how to carry his load, but the load would never be
as heavy as if he carried it alone. In time, the now infertile soil
would bear fruit.

Beginning teachers—all teachers for that matter—need
mentors. Without them we stumble and fall as we try to walk
the path. My own experience as a beginning teacher was not

without its pitfalls and crooked furrows. Even though I was well trained to teach specific strategies as a learning disabilities teacher, I was easily distracted by what seemed new and innovative as a teaching technique. I had no one to pull me back on track, no one to carry the load for me as I learned my way. The amount of paperwork in itself was enough to cause me to lose my focus and forget where I was going.

It would have been wonderful to have someone wiser and more experienced to come alongside and show me the way. As the years went by, I did find teachers who became the mentors I longed for. But at times even they fell short, and I found myself discouraged and disillusioned. Part of the problem was that we weren't headed for the same destination. My values as a Christian teacher and theirs didn't quite match. A tug-of-war ensued instead, and the yoke broke.

As far as humans go, we can have different companions for different journeys. When my goal was to become acclimated to my new school, a seasoned veteran, well liked by the principal, became my partner. When my goal was to find a way to reach gifted children with learning disabilities, my university professor from my master's program walked that road with me. And when I struggled to discover the key to motivating my students from the inside out, I needed someone who believed the way I did about how the heart and soul operate this side of heaven.

As much as we try to find a good match, we often are unequally yoked. No one can compare to how perfectly God fits our strengths and weaknesses, our desires and fears, our gifts and our talents. He is the perfect partner. Being yoked to Him shows us how our burdens are meant to be carried—with Him doing the brunt of the work.

Beasts of Burden

An animal such as a donkey or an ox used to carry or pull things or do other heavy work. The image of a donkey or an ox was familiar in biblical times. They are mentioned throughout Scripture. I envision the mother of our Lord riding a donkey into Bethlehem while she carried Him before His birth. We see a donkey used in the story of the Good Samaritan when he took the injured man to an inn to be cared for. Then we see our Lord Himself request the services of a donkey set aside for this very purpose upon His arrival at Jerusalem before He was given up to death. It doesn't seem to be a bad thing to be a beast of burden. It appears to be an honor to do the Lord's work and be created for that very purpose.

If we feel the heaviness of the Lord's call on our backs and are struggling to break free of this weight, we're probably not aware of the fact that each of us is designed to carry the load we're given. Each duty, each task, set before us as a teacher can seem burdensome. But it's when we pick up and carry more than our share that we feel our backs breaking. In two illustrations above, we see the donkey is carrying the Lord Himself. His load is light in comparison to what we find ourselves carrying each day. The weight of God's glory is not nearly as cumbersome as the weight of our own glory.

When they approached Jerusalem and came to Bethphage at the Mount of Olives, Jesus then sent two disciples, telling them, "Go into the village ahead of you. At once you will find a donkey tied there, and a colt with her. Untie them and bring them to Me. If anyone says anything to you, you should say that the Lord needs them, and immediately he will send them." (Matt. 21:1–3)

The Lord needs you! He has sent for you, and you are uniquely prepared to carry the weight of His glory. You experience stress and strain when you choose to carry the overbearing weight of your own glory. As a teacher, called to educate the minds and hearts of children, you can easily lose that eternal perspective and become focused instead on your own successes and failures with students. You begin to pick up excess baggage, such as faulty philosophies, political agendas, societal expectations, and peer pressure. This baggage is like adding rocks to your pack along a hike and will eventually pull you off balance and cause you to stumble. You'll become consumed with how heavy the pack is and lose sight of your destination.

Yoke of Purpose

Is there a purpose behind being yoked? God chooses the yoke that will help align you to His will and better serve His purposes. No matter what you believe, the truth is that you are always yoked to someone or something. What causes you to turn this way and that? Is it the world or your heavenly Master?

YOKE OF OPPRESSION

Throughout history God's people have endured the cruel yokes of oppression, the perfecting yokes of trial and tribulation, and the yoke of slavery. Our natural tendency is to seek release from these yokes. Yet we are tied to them, and they appear inescapable. My own experience as a teacher has shown me the extent of an uncomfortable and unwelcome yoke. Not every regular education teacher welcomed me, a new special education teacher, into their midst my first year of teaching. By the end of that first year, the yoke of oppression weighed heavily on my shoulders. My idealistic attitude was the only thing that held me up during periodic assaults on my program and students. The lack of support and outward expressions of disdain threatened to break my spirit. I thought it was up to me to change the hearts and minds of those teachers who seemed to disapprove of my calling to teach children who learned "differently."

More than once during my career, I felt the yoke of oppression. I've cried to the Lord to remove this heavy yoke from my neck. But I discovered my obsession with changing the minds of others to like me and the children I taught is what made that yoke heavy. It wasn't my job to change their hearts. I had taken on a burden that wasn't mine to carry. The yoke of oppression is a reality. But I can carry it as long as I don't add to its weight with unrealistic expectations, misplaced loyalties, or misguided attempts for approval.

YOKE OF TRIAL AND TRIBULATION

Sometimes the yoke you're bound to is intended to perfect your faith. It's so tempting to avoid that. It can be frightening, tiring, and tempting all at the same time. It may feel like persecution. It may feel as barren as the desert wilderness. Yet it's as necessary for your spiritual well-being as water is for your physical body.

At these times, you're misunderstood, your motives are mistaken, your friends stand aloof, and it feels as if enemies seek your life, trying to destroy your credibility and effectiveness. These are the times to be still and not fidget in a frenzy. Have you ever taught in a situation in which you felt unappreciated, unwelcome, or unsafe? Your knee-jerk reaction may be to transfer and get out from under the trial. Often younger teachers are less willing to stay and endure the trial at hand. The burnout time for new teachers is now three years! Consider the following:

> *The LORD is good to those who wait for Him,*
> *to the person who seeks Him.*

> *It is good to wait quietly*
> *for deliverance from the LORD.*
> *It is good for a man to bear the yoke*
> *while he is still young. (Lam. 3:25–27)*

Consider the wisdom offered by Bible commentator Matthew Henry:

> Afflictions do and will work very much for good: many
> have found it good to bear this yoke in their youth; it
> has made many humble and serious, and has weaned
> them from the world, who otherwise would have been
> proud and unruly. If tribulation work patience, that
> patience will work experience, and that experience a
> hope that makes not ashamed. Due thoughts of the
> evil of sin, and of our own sinfulness, will convince us
> that it is of the Lord's mercies we are not consumed.
> If we cannot say with unwavering voice, The Lord is
> my portion; may we not say, I desire to have Him for
> my portion and salvation, and in His word do I hope?
> Happy shall we be, if we learn to receive affliction as
> laid upon us by the hand of God.

Young teachers will do well to learn how to endure affliction and allow God to work in their lives. They must learn at some point to trust God and believe He knows what He's doing and where He's going. The sooner they do that, the more effective they will be in their work.

YOKE OF SLAVERY

Images of slaves yoked together while herded to a new location flicker through my mind when I think of this yoke. Although most likely none of you are literal slaves to a master, you may be servant to your students, parents, administrators, and tax payers in society. You all serve various "masters" during your lives. That particular yoke may feel quite heavy and threaten to break you because it's frustrating to feel as if everyone is your boss. But you're called to serve them well.

All who are under the yoke as slaves must regard their own masters to be worthy of all respect, so that God's name and His teaching will not be blasphemed. And those who have believing masters should not be disrespectful to them because they are brothers, but should serve them better, since those who benefit from their service are believers and dearly loved. Teach and encourage these things. (1 Tim. 6:1–2)

The Lord said no one can serve two masters. If you choose to serve Christ first, you'll be yoked to Him. This doesn't mean you don't have to submit to the authority of principals. But it does mean you'll be better able to serve them in a way that doesn't slander the name of the Lord.

The older and more experienced teacher must teach this truth to the younger, beginning teacher. It's a necessary part of the mentoring process. It can be disillusioning for a new teacher to discover that she's not in as much control of her classroom and students as she thought she'd be. Others are in control, and they tend to make decisions about how to run our classrooms without consulting teachers. How teachers respond to that discovery can ultimately determine success or failure as a teacher. One way or the other, we are slaves. But we can choose to exchange the yoke of man's bondage for Christ's.

Lighten Your Load

Those burdensome rocks we pick up along our way weigh us down. We become desperate for rest early in our careers because we're carrying more than we should. In 1990, it was estimated teachers reach burnout in approximately seven years.

The results of a 2003 National Center for Education survey, released in August 2004, said teachers reach burnout in an unbelievable and disturbing two and a half years! New teachers don't stay long enough to really know what they're doing. In my experience, the first year was full of excitement but also trepidation. The second year was familiar, but I was still working out the bugs of curriculum and teaching strategies. The third year was the charm! Too many teachers don't make it to the third year. Why? Disillusionment and an overwhelming workload chase them out the door.

There are many responsibilities you can't escape as a teacher, but you can leave some things at the wayside, both physically and philosophically.

- Love students without becoming their parents. Be more like a grandparent who can love students when they're with them but give them back to the parents at the end of the day.
- Don't say yes to extra duties unless you have honestly considered the impact they will have on your students, planning time, energy level, and family time.
- Become a learner of your students and not of the state test.
- Plan now or pay later.
- Help a teacher in need now before his problem grows and affects others later.
- Simplify, simplify, simplify! Look for ways to streamline your teaching day.

Your job is to do everything heartily as unto the Lord—unto the Lord, not unto your principal. If you focus on pleasing the Lord with the work of your hands, you'll please man as well. The burden of pleasing the Lord is infinitely lighter than trying to please man.

God never expected you to walk this path alone. When you believe in Christ, you're yoked to Him by the Holy Spirit. The Spirit gently prods you in the way to go. He will never lead you astray. But you have to welcome that yoke like the hand of a good friend, someone you trust to walk alongside you. Sometimes that yoke manifests itself in a veteran teacher whose faith matches yours and who shares the same destination. Sometimes it's the reproof of an administrator to nudge you back to the proper educational path. And if you walk away from the path like an obstinate mule, sometimes the Spirit takes drastic measures to hurry you back to the safety of the carefully plowed furrow. You see, Christ already walked the path before you, removed the rocks that would hinder you, and softened the soil beneath your feet. You can trust His leading. He's already carrying the brunt of the burdens. All you have to do is follow.

Rest Stops
Replace what is missing from your depleted diet with vitamin and mineral supplements.

Rest Reminders
Trust in the LORD with all your heart,
and do not rely on your own understanding;
think about Him in all your ways,
and He will guide you on the right paths.
PROVERBS 3:5–6

When we are tired, we are attacked
by ideas we conquered long ago.
FRIEDRICH NIETZSCHE

Journal Prompt

Whomever or whatever you're yoked to determines your steps. What's turning your head this way and that? Can you recognize what and whom God is using in your life to steer you in the right direction?

Chapter Six

Renewal of Spirit

God, create a clean heart for me
and renew a steadfast spirit within me.
PSALM 51:10

TO ME THE PROCESS of learning to read is magical. Not only does an individual finally connect the truth that symbols written on a page have sound and meaning attached, but a world beyond his imagination opens its door and changes the person forever. As a teacher of children with reading problems and then later as a parent, I experienced joy and excitement watching a child make these extraordinary connections. It's like what I felt when my son took his first steps. I knew it was nothing I did. He was ready. His body was ready. He knew he could do it. He wanted to do it. And he did.

As teachers we watch in wonder when a child finally "gets it." When a difficult concept is mastered or a confusing idea is suddenly clarified, we celebrate with the student (if only on the inside). An emerging reader must first *believe* that what's on the page is either important or interesting to know before he's motivated to think about the sounds the letters make and finally combines them in a meaningful way into words, sentences, and stories. Students move from emerging readers and writers to developing readers and writers and finally to fluent readers and writers. As we journey toward rest and renewal, we must first *believe* they are important and can be found.

There is an undeniable connection between spirit, mind, and body. What we *believe* to be true will become what we *think* and finally how we *act*. What we *do* is a direct reflection of what we *believe*. But believing comes first. For Christians, the renewing of our minds and lives cannot happen unless we first believe. In order for us to change how and if we find rest and renewal, we must first examine what we believe.

As educators you're used to making comparisons in order to clarify a concept. If your goal is to enter into rest, find out what that looks like. If you're a fluent reader, you read and understand quickly and with a minimum of effort. Similarly, a fluent "rester" is someone who can enter into rest quickly and with minimum effort. Jesus said, "Remain in Me," as if it's easy to do. What gets in your way? Usually faulty beliefs are the obstacles.

• *Rest is something I have to prepare myself for.*

Rest is not something you create for yourself. Rest is something God created for you. You don't have to be perfect to enter into His rest. You merely have to be willing. Sometimes beginning teachers believe every moment must be accounted for. Planning periods are for planning. Christmas and Easter breaks are for catching up. And summer is for working a second job to make ends meet. Teaching is one of the only jobs in America that doesn't allow for real breaks. When I worked as an administrative assistant, I discovered that every few hours I was allocated a ten-minute break and every day I was given an hour for lunch. It was stipulated by the union. It was nonnegotiable. Teachers don't have such luxuries.

I used to think the only way I could rest was to finish all my work before leaving school. When I got home, I could finally rest. If I wanted my full thirty minutes for a peaceful lunch, I had to make sure I'd already checked my mailbox, returned parent phone calls, and prepared for the class after lunch. I had to get ready for rest! Needless to say, it never happened. Believing that you must prepare in order to actually find rest is not true.

- *Rest is something the lazy do.*

We are admonished not to eat the bread of idleness. But rest and idleness (or laziness) are two different things. God Himself rested on the seventh day. Would we say He was lazy? Even the omnipresent, omniscient, omnipotent God of the universe chose to rest. We are all busy. Is it any wonder since we are created in His image?

I have to admit I stole disapproving glances at teachers who actually sat in the teachers lounge laughing and enjoying their meal, while I sat at my desk gulping down my tuna sandwich and grading papers. How could they have nothing to do? How could they possibly have time to enjoy themselves? It was beyond my comprehension and my experience.

The more comfortable and capable I became in my job, the more easily I found ways to relax and, yes, even laugh a little. God didn't rest because He didn't have anything else to do. He rested because it, too, was *good*. He modeled for us to stop, even if it's in the middle of something, and rest. It's not quitting. It's not laziness. It's created by God, and it's good.

- *I don't know how to sit still.*

King Solomon compared all that we pursue, all that we spend our time doing, and all that we desire to chasing the wind. Some of us flit from activity to activity as if we're indeed being chased. Teachers are busy people with more than their share of work, and I've seen many teachers never sit still. It's not necessarily how much work they have to do, since we all have about the same mile-high pile of paperwork. It's more about how they do that work that wears someone out just watching them. There's a difference between eating a meal and a feeding frenzy. A frenetic pace is tiring.

I shared office space one year with an itinerant teacher. For her personality, the itinerant position suited. She was what I fondly call a "hummingbird" teacher. She thrived, flitting from place to place and task to task. And she consumed more than her share of sugar and caffeine to maintain that pace. Getting her to sit still for even the briefest conversation was like trying to cage a wild hummingbird.

This didn't mean Janey didn't require rest. In fact, she craved it. Teachers are birds of a feather. We all do about the same job. We all have about the same demands on our time. We all have the same twenty-four hours in order to complete the tasks before us. Rest doesn't have to be declared as a state of emergency. Rest is something we either believe is important, or not. Janey couldn't find rest because she didn't believe it really could be found.

What Should You Believe?

The truth about rest is that you can't find it without God. It's God-created and God-ordained for His purposes and yours. When you're troubled, you become restless.

> *Hamath and Arpad are put to shame,*
> *for they have heard a bad report and are agitated;*
> *in the sea there is anxiety that cannot be calmed.*
> *Damascus has become weak;*
> *she has turned to run;*
> *panic has gripped her.*
> *Distress and labor pains have seized her*
> *like a woman in labor. (Jer. 49:23–24)*

Although this passage is talking about cities, the cities were full of people, and these people were troubled and disheartened. Have you ever felt restless as a teacher? Have you been disheartened, troubled, and tempted to flee? Did you ask for a transfer to another school, based on emotion and not career advancement? Have you considered quitting teaching altogether because you're discouraged?

Your restlessness is just what the Enemy will use to move you away from where God intends you to do good. Satan knows the powerful position in which God has placed you. The best defense if you're restless is to meditate on the truth.

- *God will protect you so you can rest.*

> *I keep the LORD in mind always.*
> *Because He is at my right hand,*
> *I will not be shaken.*
> *Therefore my heart is glad,*
> *and my spirit rejoices;*
> *my body also rests securely.*
> *For You will not abandon me to Sheol;*
> *You will not allow Your Faithful One to see the Pit.*
> *(Ps. 16:8–10)*

When I taught in Florida, tornado watches and warnings were common. We routinely conducted "duck and cover" drills with our students. One year I taught in a portable classroom. If there was a tornado warning, I was supposed to take my students to the main building for safety. Our classroom was very much like a mobile home and therefore a tornado magnet! A *watch* meant conditions were conducive to tornado activity and we should take precautions. A *warning* meant the tornado was heading our way and we should take cover! Either way, the main building was a tornado shelter, and it would have been foolish and dangerous not to run to it.

Do you believe God is your shelter from the storm? There is a way to find rest, even in the midst of a terrible storm. Have you ever noticed how babies and toddlers can sleep in their parents' arms even through a severe thunder and lightning storm? They rest comfortably and peacefully because they know they're safe. You can know that same peace even while the winds of your tornadolike life swirl around. Run under the shelter of God's wings, for there you'll find both safety and rest. Don't stand out in the rain and wonder why you're getting wet. Whether it's a watch or a warning, seek shelter.

- *God is the One who restores you to rest.*
  Do not banish me from Your presence
  or take Your Holy Spirit from me.
  Restore the joy of Your salvation to me,
  and give me a willing spirit.
  Then I will teach the rebellious Your ways,
  and sinners will return to You. (Ps. 51:11–13)

The beginning teacher is the picture of idealism. Her enthusiasm inspires some but sickens others. Veteran teachers know too well how unrealistic the expectations of a first-year teacher are. Eventually, though, everything breaks down. You can be the most organized, most focused teacher, and sooner or later things fall apart. It's the nature of the universe. Little by little you forget why you went into teaching in the first place, and slowly but surely your job becomes more like forced labor than an inspired calling. Unfortunately, your lack of enthusiasm paints a poor picture of teaching to those considering the field. It hinders the cause of teaching. Who would want to join the ranks of such a discouraged and at times disgruntled bunch?

Faith is like that. You come to it with enthusiasm, great joy, and even greater expectations. Then slowly but surely you lose momentum. You begin to look outside yourself for ways to stay motivated and to keep the faith. You sign up for Bible studies, retreats, and Sunday school classes to learn more about what you believe and to stay on track. You serve in ministries, tithe regularly, and fellowship with others just like you to let the world see what you believe. But you're tired—oh, so tired—and it's starting to show. You become disheartened or disillusioned and act in ways "unbecoming" a Christian as a result. This can hinder the cause of Christ. Instead of a sweet aroma, you exude a repellent odor.

> *Restore the joy of Your salvation to me,*
> *and give me a willing spirit. (v. 12)*

Restoration lies not in what you do to keep yourself motivated. It lies in the saving work of Christ alone. The beginner and finisher of your faith is Christ. He can restore to you the joy of salvation. But it's the willing spirit that will sustain that joy. God can grant that as well. As you pray for rest and renewal, pray that the Lord will indeed restore your joy and grant you a willing spirit. Then trust that He has done it.

- *Rest is found in God alone.*

> *I am at rest in God alone;*
> *my salvation comes from Him.*
> *He alone is my rock and my salvation,*
> *my stronghold; I will never be shaken. (Ps. 62:1–2)*

David spent a lot of time running and hiding from his enemies. During that time it must have been difficult to lay his head down and rest peacefully. Most likely his sleep was fitful and continually disturbed. David knew he was living in a state of chaos and fear. He went to the only real source of rest—rest he could count on even during only the briefest and most restless sleep. When you're tired, your spirit, mind, and body are in a weakened state. You're not at your best, and your decision making can be faulty. Your reflexes are sluggish, and your emotions run high. You worry about many things beyond your control.

There were nights filled with nightmares during the time I taught severely learning disabled students in the projects of Tampa, Florida. I worried about both the present and the future of my students. Some of them might not survive to age eighteen. Some might not survive the night—and there was nothing I could do about it. How could I rest when my thoughts and prayers were consumed with worry? I could go to the only real source for rest. God the Father knew each of my students by name and could count the hairs on each of their heads. He loved them more than I ever could and had a bigger stake in their future than I could imagine. I had to trust that. If I didn't, I didn't really believe about God what I said I believed. Restlessness can turn to rest only when we believe in the source of rest.

Snuggle up under the shelter of His wings. Believe that God is the only One who can attend to your burdens and provide you with a safe haven. He waits for you to come and be refreshed.

Rest Stops

Don't wait until you retire to be spontaneous. Build spontaneity into your overscheduled life by taking a day off and going somewhere you've never been before, or just snuggle up with your favorite book in a well-shaded hammock in your own backyard.

Rest Reminders

For You have made me rejoice, LORD,
by what You have done;
I will shout for joy
because of the works of Your hands.
PSALM 92:4

Peace is a necessary condition of spirituality,
no less than an inevitable result of it.
ALDOUS HUXLEY

Journal Prompt

Examine your beliefs about rest. Can you identify
faulty thinking? How has that faulty thinking hindered
you from entering into God's rest?

Chapter Seven
Renewal of Mind

Do not be conformed to this age, but be transformed by the renewing of your mind, so that you may discern what is the good, pleasing, and perfect will of God.
ROMANS 12:2

HOW PEOPLE THINK is the subject of much research. Why? Because people act on what they think, and if they can change how they think, they can change how they act. Teachers are always encouraging students to become active learners—those who take responsibility for their own learning and make positive choices. Since many of them don't *think* about their learning, teachers look for ways to *change their minds*.

Think back to your education as a teacher. How many workshops or seminars did you attend that focused on thinking skills or tools, habits of mind, or critical thinking? It's true that before you can change your ways, you must first change your mind. Living in this fallen world, we have developed bad habits of mind. We can change those habits of thinking and be transformed. The first step is to believe what you hear is true. At this point belief is the catalyst for real, life-altering change. Without it, an exercise in developing better thinking habits is futile.

How can we sift what we hear in a seminar on thinking skills through the Word of God? In order for us, as teachers, to make a lasting impact on students, we must pattern our thinking on God's. First, let's assess some current thinking on thought and see if it stands up under the scrutiny of God's truth.

Popular inspirational speaker and author Robert J. Marzano defines habits of mind as mental habits individuals can develop to render their thinking and learning more self-regulated. These mental habits include:

- Being aware of your own thinking
- Planning
- Being aware of necessary resources
- Being sensitive to feedback
- Evaluating the effectiveness of your actions[3]

We could analyze many other schools of thought on thinking, but let's use Marzano's to see if his philosophy lines up with God's Word.

- *Being aware of your own thinking*
  The heart is more deceitful than anything else
  and desperately sick—who can understand it?
  I, the LORD, examine the mind,
  I test the heart
  to give to each according to his way,
  according to what his actions deserve. (Jer. 17:9–10)

Sometimes how you think is really a collection of habits. You can fool yourself into thinking things that aren't true about yourself, others, and situations. You make assumptions about why others behave the way they do and draw conclusions based on those assumptions. You feed misconceptions with your own fears and build them into lies. Your interactions with students and their parents can at times contribute to a budding defensive mind-set. Bitterness takes root, and its deadly tendrils wrap around your heart.

These bad habits of thought then determine how you approach every new relationship with students or parents. It's difficult to recognize them because these thoughts are masked by your own sinful nature. God is the only one who can see them for what they truly are and completely remove the bitter root. Pray that He will reveal them to you, so that you can replace the lies with His truth. Then you'll be able to see students and their parents as God does and be able to serve their needs with His love.

- *Planning*

For God is not unjust; He will not forget your work and the love you showed for His name when you served the saints—and you continue to serve them. Now we want each of you to demonstrate the same diligence for the final realization of your hope, so that you won't become lazy, but imitators of those who inherit the promises through faith and perseverance. (Heb. 6:10–12)

God doesn't dissuade you from planning. In fact, He counts on it. With due diligence you must persevere in your desire to serve Him. Examine those who are doing what you hope to do and pattern your life after theirs. When you knew you wanted to be a teacher, you found out how others became what you wanted to become and you followed their lead. Your hope became your plan.

- *Being aware of necessary resources*

According to the grace given to us, we have different gifts: If prophecy, use it according to the standard of faith; if service, in service; if teaching, in teaching; if exhorting, in exhortation; giving, with generosity; leading, with diligence; showing mercy, with cheerfulness. (Rom. 12:6–8)

As you have been given gifts to serve the kingdom, so have others who work with you—so have the students and parents you serve. As you ponder what to do next, consider those gifts and see how you can tap into them to accomplish the work God has given you, in a way that's pleasing to Him.

- *Being sensitive to feedback*

> *Do not despise the LORD's instruction, my son,*
> *and do not loathe His discipline;*
> *for the LORD disciplines the one He loves,*
> *just as a father, the son he delights in. (Prov. 3:11–12)*

You seem to get feedback from a variety of sources, some within the education community and some without. Everyone tells you how to do your job better. Everyone seems to be your boss. And each year your annual evaluation is put into writing and sequestered in a file in the district office. How you respond to feedback tells a lot about who you think you are. Be someone your Father delights in!

- *Evaluating the effectiveness of your actions*

> *For by the grace given to me, I tell everyone among you not*
> *to think of himself more highly than he should think. Instead,*
> *think **sensibly,** as God has distributed a measure of faith to*
> *each one. (Rom. 12:3, emphasis added)*

How do you know when you're successful? By the percentage of students who achieve higher than a C in your class? Or by the measurable improvement they make on the state test? By how well behaved your students are or how talented? No. Success is measured by how much glory you bring to God. Glory is not about you. It's only about God and belongs only to God. Whatever you gain, whatever praises you receive as an educator, all belong to God. Take a long, hard look at how you do what you do. Consider it all in the light of God's glory. Only then will you know how well you're doing.

Take Every Thought Captive

We demolish arguments and every high-minded thing that is raised up against the knowledge of God, taking every thought captive to the obedience of Christ. (2 Cor. 10:4b–5)

At times your thoughts are in rebellion to Christ. They control your actions in ways contrary to God's truth and principles. It may seem, on the surface, like the tail is wagging the dog.

But you can turn this around and take these thoughts captive without mercy. Bind them and replace them with godly thinking instead. You're challenged to do this every day in school. Look at it as plenty of opportunities to practice thinking God's way.

Some Thoughts to Think About

Here are common thoughts that begin as simple observations, but then take root and may control how you treat others. They are not from God. They are from the Enemy, and they must be captured and bound.

- *No one appreciates what I do.* If you never receive a thank-you note from a parent, a gift from a student, a pat on the back from your principal, or a show of support from your family, you may be underappreciated. But when that thought—which easily breezes in and out of your mind—decides to take up residence, it begins to dictate how you react to parents, how you respond to students, how you respect your principal, and how you rely on your family. You begin to back away and shut down. No rest is found in the company of this thought—only inner turmoil.

- *I'm all alone in this.* Teaching can be quite isolating by its nature—one teacher in a classroom with students. Some beginning teachers cite this as the most disturbing discovery their first year. Thoughts of isolation can quickly turn into actions of self-preservation. You think you're alone, so you act as if you are. Community breaks down when the walls of isolation go up. Relationships wither and die. You can't reach the hearts and minds of others from behind a brick wall. Don't allow this thought to determine your interaction at school. You are all a part of one body. Don't cut yourself off!

- *Parents just don't get it.* Most parents *don't* know what your life is like as a teacher. They're concerned about how you interact with their children, and on that level they can be very child-centered. But parents can understand what your life is like if you share it with them. This doesn't mean whine and complain to them, but you can educate parents about the reality of how things work at school. Engage in enough of a relationship so they can see your struggles, and maybe, if you let them, they can help. You may be the education "expert," but you're not the only one. Parents are the experts on their children. You could learn a thing or two.

  This way of thinking will only isolate you further from those you need to reach and teach. Corral it and cripple its effect on your life and your teaching.

- *Students are apathetic.* Many certainly may be that. But not all students are apathetic. And those who are, are not apathetic *all* the time. If you categorize students in this way, you don't allow room for growth, maturity, or passion. It's a thought that excuses you from tending to their needs because you think it won't matter. Be grateful God didn't make His decisions based on whether or not you're passionate about Him.

*But God proves His own love for us in that while we were
still sinners Christ died for us! (Rom. 5:8)*

This thinking will only separate you from those you
came to serve. Love them in spite of their apathy and
receive reconciliation. Reconciliation brings peace.

If you're not careful, you can think yourself right out of a
job. Perception is everything. You are what you think. Make sure
you sift each thought through God's sieve. His wisdom is the
only way that brings life and peace.

Rest Stops

Learn how to say no and delete many of the "shoulds" from
your life.

Rest Reminders

"Martha, Martha, you are worried and upset about many
things, but one thing is necessary. Mary has made the right
choice, and it will not be taken away from her."
LUKE 10:41B–42

Meditation and prayer are to the soul what reflection,
study, and conversation are to the mind and what exercise,
physical work, and sports are to the body.
ANONYMOUS

Journal Prompt

Have you found yourself thinking some things that are
not true? Capture and bind those thoughts! Don't wait.
The sooner you rid yourself of them, the sooner you
can replace them with godly thinking.

Chapter Eight

Renewal of Body

Youths may faint and grow weary, and young men stumble
and fall, but those who trust in the LORD will renew their
strength; they will soar on wings like eagles; they will run
and not grow weary; they will walk and not faint.

ISAIAH 40:30–31

THE FIREWORKS EXPLODED all around me as I sat in
complete tranquillity in a home in the town of my birth. Not
only was New York Harbor host to a spectacular display of this
country's independence, it echoed the independent thinking
and actions our forefathers took more than two hundred years
ago. Their thoughts of a nation independent of the rule of a king
turned into actions that secured our current way of life—the
kind of life people flock to from every corner of the planet.

The actions we take while in the body reveal to a watching
world what we value and what we believe to be true. Our
choices, lived out in our day-to-day lives, require our attention
before we can ever hope to find rest.

I wonder sometimes if the choices I've made over the
years—the ones that seemed in defiance of the status quo, the
ones no one else seemed to understand—attracted followers.
Independent thinking characterized my youth, shaped my present, and will mark my future. I think my choices aren't the

attraction, but my own reaction to them either attracts or repels others. Often my choices caused me more work, more anxiety, and less peace. I doubt if anyone would want to pattern her life after mine in that case. But in following the path less traveled, there can still be peace. In following an independent spirit, there can be rest. The key is in the conviction that my actions can be traced back to whom I was following. The phrase "take me to your leader" is much more than a line in a science fiction B movie.

I chose a different path when I chose special education as a major in college. I chose a different path when I pursued a master's degree in gifted education and taught middle school gifted children. I chose a different path when I left teaching for a time to stay home with my babies. I chose yet another path when I decided to homeschool our two children for five years. Many people in my life shook their heads in dismay when I walked these paths. The difference between these choices and ones I made earlier in my life to be "independent" was that I was following a *king* and not my own independent thinking. Our forefathers probably would shake their heads at me as well.

Keeping in mind the previous discussions of how what you believe shapes what you think and spurs you to action, examine your actions. Consider these elements of the path you walk as an educator and whether they reflect your belief in the King.

Choosing a Teaching Position

I wanted to make a difference. That was what drove me to declare myself an education major during my freshman year of college. Choosing what to teach was a different story. I wavered and waffled between elementary education, secondary education, Latin, and children with special needs. Everyone I talked to had a very strong opinion about which would be best. I got the distinct feeling that choosing one meant rejecting another. I hope the atmosphere in the colleges of education at major universities has changed; but then there was a definite line in the sand, and college students had to choose sides.

Inside, I knew where God was calling me, but it wasn't easy to ignore peer pressure. I knew my choice was not the popular choice. I knew my classics professors would be disappointed in me. Yet I chose special education anyway. The special education department at my college was not as well organized as the elementary or secondary programs. We special ed majors were not tracked together throughout the years. We didn't spend time together learning how to act as a team. Our program was designed to help us learn how to meet the unique, individual needs of students, so we functioned as individuals and not teams as the regular education students did. It served its purpose, but I remember feeling separated and isolated within my own college.

Drawing on many factors, you choose what to teach and which kinds of students to serve; but nothing is by accident, and you are where God calls you to be. Even if you find yourself in a department that was not your first choice, it isn't a mistake. Nothing is wasted. God redeems all. He makes everything work together for His good purposes. Twenty years later I find myself about to teach high school Latin! It means adding a subject to my certification. It means changing my lifestyle completely. It means trusting God to complete the good work He started in me all those years ago.

Your choice to teach in the first place is a response to God's calling. Whether you heeded the whispering call of His still, small voice or finally responded to the Holy Spirit taking you by the shoulders and redirecting your path, you are right where you belong. Rest in that!

How to Treat Others

I spend a lot of time sharing with people why teachers are discouraged and at times brokenhearted. As I attempt to connect relevance to their lives, I say, "When you're really discouraged or frustrated, do you do a good job?" My goal is to make the case that they should all encourage and support their children's teachers. They should nurture relationships with teachers so they in turn are better able to nurture children. As much as I believe in the encouragement of teachers, I also believe teachers can do a good job, one that is glorifying to God regardless of whether anyone ever says, "Good job!" to them.

You've heard the adage "If Momma ain't happy, ain't nobody happy." The same can be said of teachers: If the teacher ain't (isn't) happy, ain't none of her students happy. This is a powerful statement. On the one hand, it reveals the power a teacher has over his students. It also reveals whose responsibility it is to control his own behavior so that it doesn't adversely affect his students. What a sobering thought!

It's not up to my students to make me feel good about myself so I can then treat them well. It's up to me as a follower of Christ to exhibit the character of God in how I treat my students. The fruits of the Spirit (Gal. 5:22–26) are what I pray will flow from me into the lives of those in my charge. Not only will my students benefit from the life-giving power of these fruits, but so will their parents, my colleagues, and those in authority over me.

- *Love:* Christ's love within you can flow out to everyone you touch in your school. Love when you don't want to. Love your enemies. Love so that they know the God you serve.
- *Joy:* Share the joy of the Lord with those around you regardless of whether your students do well on a state

test, whether a behavior problem is resolved, or whether you get a sufficient pay raise. The joy of your salvation emanates throughout all circumstances—happy, sad, or indifferent.

- *Peace:* Again, peace is not dependent on circumstances. You can experience God's peace in the midst of a whirlwind. But it's also the peace you can give others when turmoil cries for your attention—peace when you're dealing with a difficult student, when you're conferencing with a belligerent parent, and when you're relating to an arrogant colleague or administrator.

- *Patience:* One of the greatest attributes a teacher can have is patience. Patience comes when you trust the Lord for the outcome. Patience while you wait for a student to finally get it. Patience while you wait for a society to appreciate you. Patience while a difficult situation moves toward resolution.

- *Kindness:* Kindness reveals its strength when you extend compassion and benevolence toward those least deserving. You can be kind in the face of a furious parent, kind to a reporter who slams your school in the newspaper, kind when a colleague talks negatively about you behind your back.

- *Goodness:* Doing what is right even in the face of wrong characterizes goodness. It's good to be honest about a child's performance even when your principal encourages you to do otherwise. It's good to give your administrator the respect of his or her position even if he or she doesn't respect yours as a teacher. It's good to fill out every required documentation of student progress even if you disagree with its use.

- *Faith:* This faith is not in a person, a system, or a teaching strategy. It's faith in the living God who requires it even amid undeniable obstacles, confidence that God will work all your experiences in school together for His good purposes, assurance that you serve the God of the universe and that nothing is wasted in that service, and reliance on God to fulfill your every need, even when your budget is meager and your support missing.
- *Gentleness:* A gentle spirit is not easily ruffled. It's the fruit you most need to cultivate the rest you seek. A gentle tongue is one that speaks the truth in love. A gentle hand is one that eases another with a soft touch. A gentle attitude brings calm to a stormy situation.
- *Self-control:* Be diligent to cultivate these fruits. The Holy Spirit works in concert with your will to bring about change within you and produce these fruits. Show restraint by avoiding occasions for sin. Practice self-discipline as you break old habits and build new ones. You can exercise strength of mind and will as you focus on the things above by not worrying about what you can't change about students, their parents, or their upbringing.

The fruits of the Spirit produce rest and renewal by their very existence. The gardener toils in order to be able to rest under the shade of his trees and later enjoy the fruit of his labor. You toil day after day, but rest won't come if you aren't doing what it takes to produce fruit.

How to Treat Your Family

Teaching can be an all-consuming job. Good teachers know that nothing less than 100 percent will get the job done. Great teachers give 110 percent! Teachers with families find themselves torn as they try to balance competing demands. I've heard that a good marriage is when each partner gives 50 percent. The truth is each partner must give 100 percent—which is mathematically impossible yet personally necessary.

Even though at home with my family is where I can be myself and my family loves me anyway, I can't take family members for granted. Why can I say no to my husband about going to a function I'd prefer to skip, but I can't tell my principal no to an extra duty that takes me away from home at night? Why can I have the patience of Job when Jason is acting up again during reading time, but I jump on my son the moment he talks out of turn at the dinner table? Why will I hunt a particular curriculum tie-in as a favor to my department head, but I put off my mother's request to find a favorite book from her childhood? The ugly truth is that I somehow believe it's more important to submit myself to my job than to my family. My desire to please my principal, my department head, and the parents of my students overrides my desire to please my family or God.

I realize much stress and unrest I've felt over the years was because of this tug-of-war. But your students and your school will benefit from attention to your family. It's crucial to get your own house in order first before trying to bring order to the one at school. The qualifications for leaders in the early church (1 Tim. 3:1–13) are also good for teachers who are leaders today.

- *Self-controlled:* The most influential fruit of the Spirit encompasses our thoughts, words, and actions.
- *Sensible:* This person pursues and exhibits wisdom in his decisions and actions.
- *Respectable:* Reputable, highly regarded, and well thought of.
- *Hospitable:* Welcoming, friendly, generous, and kind.

- *An able teacher:* Clever, talented, intelligent, and capable.
- *Gentle, not quarrelsome:* Calm, tender, and peaceful.
- *Not greedy:* Liberal, bighearted, giving, and charitable.
- *Competent manager of her own household:* She has her children under control with all dignity. According to this Scripture passage, if anyone doesn't know how to manage his own household, how will he take care of God's church? And in this case, God's children are placed in your charge as a teacher.

These are great expectations to be sure, but you must consciously attend to the needs of your own household before turning attention to your job as an educator.

How to Treat Yourself

The Lord Jesus told us to love our neighbor as ourselves. But how do we really love ourselves? We meet our most basic needs, but isn't there more to it than that? I suspect that many of you are doing just the bare minimum to get by, and I doubt the Lord commanded you to love that way. Some of you aren't even doing that. Your bodies are broken or run down. You don't eat well or get enough sleep. You keep waiting for someone to notice your need and fill it. And no one ever does. Most likely, others don't know how to love themselves either and therefore are unable to really love you the way Jesus commanded. You yourself have to love and care for the temple of the Holy Spirit the way God intended.

> *Do you not know that your body is a sanctuary of the Holy Spirit who is in you, whom you have from God? You are not your own, for you were bought at a price; therefore glorify God in your body. (1 Cor. 6:19–20)*

There are physical and chemical reasons why we may not be experiencing rest. I know my body well enough to realize that when I eat fried foods, I'm going to be up much of the night. I know sugar makes me feel sluggish during the day. I know my stomach twists in pain even with a small amount of milk in my coffee. When I don't feel good, I become restless and frustrated. The bottom line is I don't teach well when I don't feel well.

If I don't make the effort to care for my body as a good steward, then I can't expect it to perform the way I need it to. Unforeseen circumstances will crop up to either disable or dissuade me from glorifying God, but I can take care of the body God has created for me even if it becomes damaged or crippled in some way. If you've spent years abusing your body with foods, chemicals, activities, alcohol and drugs, or an unhealthy lifestyle, you can begin today, right where you are, to take care of what you still have.

You know what you ought to do and ought not do concerning your body, but it requires discipline, willpower, and restraint. It also requires forgiveness of self when you fail so you can move forward and start over again. The prize is not an athlete's physique, a model's complexion, or a nutritionist's cholesterol level. The prize is whether you've glorified God in your body—as a twenty-one-year-old first-year teacher living on macaroni and cheese, a forty-year-old career teacher wondering if her hormones will ever settle down, or a sixty-year-old veteran teacher who can't run laps with his players during practice anymore. Do the best with what you have and take great care of what you've been given.

Renewal of the body happens from the inside out. Sometimes you can look good on the outside, with every hair in place, but on the inside you've let yourself go. How you treat others is as important as how we treat yourself. Christ's commandment to love your neighbor as yourself is not only good for the neighbor but good for you. God is not glorified by a pristine appearance. He's glorified when you care for yourself and others well enough to be able to do what brings Him glory. If you can't serve Him in your present state, you have rebuilding and renovation to do!

Rest Stops
Pick up a book you've been meaning to read and allow yourself to get lost in it—finally.

Rest Reminders
Remember to dedicate the Sabbath day.
EXODUS 20:8

The body is the implement of the soul;
and the soul, of God.
PLUTARCH

Journal Prompt
What bad habits of body must you change in order to take good care of His temple? How are these habits getting in the way of finding the rest you crave?

Part 3

Learn from Me

Chapter Nine

Lord, Let Me Decrease

John responded, "No one can receive a single thing unless
it's given to him from heaven. You yourselves can testify that
I said, 'I am not the Messiah, but I've been sent ahead of
Him.' He who has the bride is the groom. But the groom's
friend, who stands by and listens for him, rejoices greatly at
the groom's voice. So this joy of mine is complete.
He must increase, but I must decrease."

JOHN 3:27–30

IT'S SO HARD SOMETIMES not to get discouraged by the
meagerness of teaching. The pay is low. The budgets continue
to shrink. The respect is dwindling to nonexistence. And the
rewards come few and far between. Maybe that's why, for some
of us, a self-preservation instinct kicks in, and we look for ways
to build ourselves up. I admit to thoughts of self-promotion and
delusions of grandeur. I even submitted my own name for
teacher of the year once! I believed I was doing a great job and
wanted to be acknowledged for it.

I've come to believe that education is all about relationship, but the evidence can be quite to the contrary. Education,
it seems, is all about image. School accountability reports, state
testing, the grading of schools, what neighborhood a school is
in, how many computers are in each classroom, how many

teachers have master's degrees or postgraduate degrees, how many have received national certification, how many championships the school's sports program has won, how many academic scholarships graduating seniors have accumulated, the graduation rate, how many grants teachers have secured for their program or school, how many honors the school has received for attendance, test scores, electricity use, PTA membership, and grounds beautification are all about image. Favorable mention in the local media is a feather in a principal's cap. Favorable mention in the national media is a crown! Glory is sought after and valued. No wonder teachers look for ways to bring glory to themselves and their own classrooms.

There is a flip side to the quest for self-validation, self-promotion, or self-preservation. We can become so self-involved we carry our worries and concerns just as closely as we carry our certificates, ribbons, plaques, and awards. This path is not only destructive, it also leads in the complete opposite direction of rest. We worry so much about obtaining and then maintaining an elite status that we forget to enjoy the bounty of God's blessings freely given. We forget why we went into teaching in the first place. We become distracted and eventually disillusioned.

Self-Validation: Who Am I?

The first man was from the earth and made of dust;
the second man is from heaven. Like the man made of dust,
so are those who are made of dust; like the heavenly man,
so are those who are heavenly. And just as we have borne
the image of the man made of dust, we will also bear the
image of the heavenly man. (1 Cor. 15:47–49)

I recently spent time going through the process of renewing my teaching certificate. At the same time I crafted a current résumé outlining who I was and what I was qualified to do as an educator. Line after line validated my expertise as a teacher, speaker, and writer. I paid fees (hefty ones!) to reinstate certain subjects on my certificate, so that when administrators look at me they will know who I am. I'm defined as someone qualified to teach exceptional student education (K–12), gifted education (K–12), educational leadership, and Latin (K–12). I am a teacher through and through. I share much with the millions of other teachers on this planet. We have a common bond. We know what one another's lives are like. We are teachers. But there's more to who I am than that.

I may bear the image of a human teacher, but as I am conformed to the image of the "heavenly man," I bear that image as well. We don't need to ignore who we were at birth. We don't need to belittle our call to be teachers either. Our focus needs to be on *becoming*. We are moving from what is natural to what is spiritual. Therein lies who we really are.

As I survey this renewed teaching certificate, I mentally add areas of certification. I am a daughter of the King. I am a bride awaiting her bridegroom. I am a precious commodity, purchased by One who paid the highest price for my life. I am of heavenly stock! What I love about this is that these declarations, although more valuable beyond reason, cost me *nothing*. The price was paid in full by Jesus Himself.

Self-Promotion: Do Not Boast of Yourself

Don't boast about tomorrow,
for you don't know what a day might bring.
Let another praise you, and not your own mouth—
a stranger, and not your own lips. (Prov. 27:1–2)

"All I have to do is open my mouth and I'll have a job," I explained to my sister. After all, during my five-year leave from teaching, I'd had numerous job offers. Each better than the last, trying to entice me to return to teaching before I was ready. Now I was ready, and I knew, with complete certainty, that my strong teaching record would secure me a much-needed job.

I was wrong.

After many phone calls I discovered to my dismay that no one was waiting for me to knock on his door announcing my triumphant return. In fact, there were no jobs to be had! My previous overconfidence turned to desperation, and I scoured the district for any job. I came up empty.

The rose-colored glasses I wore all those years ago were discarded that very day. I realized my error wasn't counting my chickens before they hatched—it was thinking I could hatch them myself.

Even now as I work to minister to other teachers, I can get caught up in the self-promotion roller coaster. This roller coaster has incredible highs, but it also promises frightening lows. My heart races up and down the hills and around the bends and turns. There is no rest on this ride. The only way to find rest is to get off.

For we don't dare classify or compare ourselves with some
who commend themselves. But in measuring themselves by
themselves and comparing themselves to themselves, they lack
understanding. We, however, will not boast beyond measure,
but according to the measure of the area of ministry that
God has assigned to us, which reaches even to you. . . .
So the one who boasts must boast in the Lord. For it is not
the one commending himself who is approved, but the one
the Lord commends. (2 Cor. 10:12–13, 17–18)

Often we compare others, their abilities, their responses, and their behaviors by our own prejudices. When we do this, we find ourselves in a more excellent position. We commend (praise) ourselves by our own standards. There is only one true measure, and that is God's Word.

The year I got my master's degree in gifted education was also the year I left exceptional education to teach sixth-grade gifted students. Very few teachers of the gifted had master's degrees. Most were merely "certified." That meant they took only three classes to qualify them to teach this population. I worked full time and went to school at night to secure this master's degree, and it started to bother me that those who chose not to complete that degree were afforded the same opportunities. I know this makes me sound extremely immature and self-centered, but at the time that's exactly what I was.

When one of these teachers made a mistake in judgment about a student's abilities or performance, I would say to someone in confidence, "They just don't know these kids the way I do. If they'd gotten their degree, they wouldn't make these kinds of mistakes." I was arrogant for a twenty-six-year-old teacher! I needed humbling.

God is good at keeping me humble. Later that year, one of the veteran gifted teachers at my school (one with a master's degree and ten years' experience) questioned my choice of semester projects. She gently suggested that it was too cumbersome for both me and my students to complete and would lead to only disappointment and frustration. I disagreed and disregarded her efforts to steer me from disaster. Only 20 percent of my students finished their projects, and I received many parent complaints about how the project was executed and the anxiety it caused children. I was devastated. How could I be so wrong? That's what happens when I compare myself only to myself!

All that matters, both in and out of the classroom, is not praising ourselves or seeking the praise of others, but whether what we do honors God. It is for His glory that we teach. It is for

His glory alone that we do the work He has prepared for our hands to do.

Self-Absorption: Focus Not on Yourself

Finally brothers, whatever is true, whatever is honorable,
whatever is just, whatever is pure, whatever is lovely,
whatever is commendable—if there is any moral excellence
and if there is any praise—dwell on these things. Do what
you have learned and received and heard and seen in me,
and the God of peace will be with you. (Phil. 4:8–9)

When we're self-absorbed, we not only focus on everything going right in our lives but also on everything going wrong. An unkind word, an unmet expectation, or an unexpected turn of events spins us into a sort of tunnel vision that blocks joy, truth, and peace. As teachers we have justifiable reasons to be disappointed, disillusioned, or discouraged. The key is not to remain in a state of disappointment, disillusionment, or discouragement. When we *focus* on something, we do it to the exclusion of everything else. We can't find rest if we don't focus on those things that lead to rest.

"Offer it up!" my mother used to say. Take those complaints, worries, and concerns, and offer them as a sacrifice of love to God. I like the upward motion of this suggestion. Once we stop looking in the mirror and look up instead, we can see those things that are true, honorable, just, pure, lovely, and commendable. Paul said to "dwell" on these things (Phil. 4:8). That doesn't mean a quick visit or a stop on the way to somewhere else. It means to reside, remain, or abide. It has a sense of permanence to it. And it's a choice.

Rest comes when we remain in God. "Remain in Me, and I in you" (John 15:4a). We can do good and produce fruit that brings glory to God only if we remain in Him.

Glory Gained: Glory to the Father, Son, and Holy Spirit

*But I have received everything in full, and I have
an abundance. I am fully supplied, having received from
Epaphroditus what you provided—a fragrant offering,
a welcome sacrifice, pleasing to God. And my God will
supply all your needs according to His riches in glory in
Christ Jesus. Now to our God and Father be glory forever
and ever. Amen. (Phil. 4:18–20)*

The apostle Paul left a life of comfort to follow Christ and spread the gospel. He was often hungry, imprisoned, and beaten for this choice, and yet he learned to be content. His comfort was in God, not in the conditions he faced day after day. He had many valid reasons to complain, but that would have led only to discontentment. Paul learned how to be content in good times and in bad. The key here is that he *learned.*

I started my teaching career in an impoverished school in the projects of Tampa, Florida. There were a host of reasons why this wasn't the ideal school for me. But somehow I was content. I learned how to do more with less and how to be grateful for this first job right out of college. I believed those students were especially chosen for me by God, and I was especially chosen to be their teacher. Later, I took a job closer to my home in a school with a bigger budget, a higher standing in the community, and a completely different population of students. I had to learn to be content all over again. It wasn't as easy this time. Even though I had more, I found I wanted more still. I squirmed uncomfortably in my pristine environment, trying to make it even better.

What makes you discontent? Pride, unbelief, a longing after something you don't have, and an aversion to what you do

have can all breed discontentment. Even under the best conditions in the best school, with the biggest budget, your own
office and phone, state-of-the-art facilities, well-behaved students, and incredible parent support, you can become discontent. Then you become restless and uncomfortable. Pray for
patience and hope when you're belittled and humility and
heavenly thoughts when praised. That's when you realize your
comfort and rest are only in God and not in circumstances.
That's why the glory is to God and to the Son and to the Holy
Spirit—and not you.

A Mathematical Improbability: Lord, Let Me Decrease

> *John responded, "No one can receive a single thing unless*
> *it's given to him from heaven. You yourselves can testify that*
> *I said, 'I am not the Messiah, but I've been sent ahead of*
> *Him.' He who has the bride is the groom. But the groom's*
> *friend, who stands by and listens for him, rejoices greatly*
> *at the groom's voice. So this joy of mine is complete. He*
> *must increase, but I must decrease." (John 3:27–30)*

No matter how well John the Baptist prophesied or how
popular he became, he knew that ultimately Jesus would
increase in honor and influence, while he himself would be followed by fewer. And he was fully satisfied with the place and
work assigned to him. That's the goal.

As a writer and speaker, I've had many opportunities to
share my love for the Lord with those who choose to listen. The
temptation for me comes when I begin to believe I must somehow increase my own name recognition in order to do the work
assigned to me. That striving, that pursuit of my own glory, only
hampers any hope of finding peace and rest. It brings with it
panic, anxiety, and worry instead.

"He likes to hear himself talk." I'm sure there is someone in your life for whom this is true. If you had to make an honest assessment, you might conclude that person is you. You must train your ears instead to listen for the groom's voice and rejoice when you hear it! Teachers are talkers. But be a listener first and foremost.

You teach to facilitate a child's learning. Children hear your voice in the classroom, but you hope that in your words, tone, and values they'll hear the voice of Jesus. If you lead them to Him, they'll follow you less and Him more. All as it should be.

You have a job to do. It's an assignment from God. In order to do it in a way that's pleasing to Him and brings Him glory, you must deny yourself, take up your cross daily, and follow Him (Luke 9:23). You become a *God*-validator, a *God*-promoter, and *God*-absorbed! Thereby you find peace.

Rest Stops
Keep your head up and smile! Some of you have to be reminded to do this. If you appear negative, you'll draw only other negative people to you. If you appear positive, you'll draw other positive people to you.

Rest Reminders
I saw that all labor and all skillful work is
due to a man's jealousy of his friend.
This too is futile and a pursuit of the wind.
The fool folds his arms
and consumes his own flesh.
Better one handful with rest,
than two handfuls with effort and pursuit of the wind.
ECCLESIASTES 4:4–6

I was too ambitious in my deed,
And thought to distance all men in success,
Till God came to me, marked the place, and said,
"Ill doer, henceforth keep within this line,
Attempting less than others"—and I stand
And work among Christ's little ones, content.
ELIZABETH BARRETT BROWNING

Journal Prompt

Have you found yourself looking for ways to improve
your image and standing at your school? It's an easy trap
to fall into. What can you do differently to become more
God-absorbed and less self-absorbed?

Chapter Ten

The Calendar of Rest

These will serve as tassels for you to look at, so that you may
remember all the LORD's commands and obey them and not
become unfaithful by following your own heart and your
own eyes. This way you will remember and obey all My
commands and be holy to your God.

NUMBERS 15:39–40

I SURVEYED THIS YEAR'S school calendar, looking for pockets of rest. A few days were scattered here and there for teacher
workdays when we wouldn't have students. A few holidays created three-day weekends, but there was nothing substantial
until Thanksgiving. I knew the fall would go fast. It always does.
It feels like a mad race to Christmas break. And then after
returning from those luxurious two weeks, we slowly march to
spring break before finishing in June.

This particular year I began with all my personal and sick
days intact. I've never been able to save my days to roll over to
the next school year as some of my colleagues boast. I have children and children get sick; therefore, I take my sick days to care
for them. So when well-meaning teachers suggest I use one day
per month strictly as a mental health day, I laugh. I guess my

mental health will just have to do without periodic and strategically placed days off.

Some teachers begin the countdown until Christmas break in September! Some begin the countdown to June the very first day of school. The school calendar is full of breaks. Quarter breaks, semester breaks, holiday breaks, and summer break become our focus.

In January, we really wonder if we will make it to spring break. Fall is full of testing and counts. Spring is saturated with even more testing and training. The school year has its ebb and flow. We start out raring to go, believing in new beginnings and great expectations. As the months go on, we collect burdens and worries that weigh heavily as we slow the pace in a funeral march to June when we should be making a proud procession to graduation.

The problem is focus. We're looking for the wrong end results. If we're to focus on the things above, we need to avert our eyes from the earthly and empty promises of the school calendar and focus instead on the life-giving calendar of the church. Many Christian churches follow a liturgical calendar to help members leave behind daily distractions and focus on what truly matters. Christmas break isn't about two weeks off from school. It's the conclusion of the Advent season and celebrating the birth of our Savior. Spring isn't about a welcome break in the middle of the semester. It's the Lenten season to contemplate Christ's death and sacrifice and to rejoice in His resurrection!

Even if you teach in a public school, you can treasure the peace and renewal the liturgical year offers. Each month may mean something practical to us as teachers, but it also can mean something spiritual. If you made a bulletin board for each month to help you stay focused, what would you put on it?

Many church calendars consist of seven seasons— Advent, Christmas, Ordinary Time, Lent, Easter Triduum, Easter, and a second Ordinary Time. Each comprises feasts, memorials, observances, and solemnities (an event in the life of Jesus and the saints). Each season points to Christ. In the busyness and urgentness of life, it helps to stop and refocus your view on what's really important. And it's not final exams, the end-of-the-year checklist, or teacher workdays. Sometimes you need reminders to separate yourself from the world, to be consecrated in order to walk through the year in obedience to God.

August: New Beginnings

Take the time this month to meditate on the pureness of Christ's love. It's without spot or blemish. His love comes new each day like a clean slate. Focus prayer time on both the practical and spiritual needs of yourself and your students.

Pray for new students, ideas to meet shrinking budget needs, your new school or position, change in daily routine, to instill respect in students from the start, and that the love of Christ will permeate your dealings with everyone.

September: Great Expectations

At this time few grades have been entered, and you have great expectations of your students and yourself. You look to stabilize your classroom routines and become better acquainted with students. Take this month to contemplate the cross of Christ. The cross of salvation brings with it great expectation of the life of the world to come. The cross comprises the passion, crucifixion, and resurrection of Christ—all in one image. Pray for the salvation of all your students.

Memorize and meditate on John 3:16. It's the meaning of the cross.

> *For God loved the world in this way: He gave His One*
> *and Only Son, so that everyone who believes in Him*
> *will not perish but have eternal life.*

October: Making the Grade

How do you measure your success as an educator? The success of your students? You do much more in the lives of children than hand out grades. You're called to be a peacemaker in the hearts of children, parents, other teachers, and those you touch in the community. Take this month to focus on what brings peace. The face of the Lord brings peace. Meditate on it. Say the prayer that Jesus Himself gave you to pray, understanding the depth of the words and how they can bring peace.

> *Our Father in heaven,*
> *Your name be honored as holy.*
> *Your kingdom come.*
> *Your will be done on earth as it is in heaven.*
> *Give us today our daily bread.*
> *And forgive us our debts,*
> *As we also have forgiven our debtors.*
> *And do not bring us into temptation,*
> *but deliver us from the evil one.*
> *[For Yours is the kingdom and the power and the glory forever.*
> *Amen.]*
> *Matthew 6:9b–13a*

November: Dying in Order to Live

With the end of fall comes a winding down, a sort of dying. In some parts of the country the leaves change colors, wither, and die. Elsewhere the grass goes dormant and the ocean waters cool. In school you feel the end of the semester coming. You begin to wrap up units and look for missing work from students so you can prepare to close the books. With endings also comes memorial. You remember what came before, knowing that you must first die before you can begin your new life in Christ.

The liturgical focus for November is commemoration of the faithful who have already departed. You remember their faithfulness, whether your own family and friends or those saints whose devotion to God are an example today. One way to do this is to visit a cemetery. Visit the graves of family members and remember how their Christian witness influenced your life. You may be surprised to discover how pleasant visiting a cemetery can be in the fall. All creation seems to be preparing to end its active life in this season to prepare for life in the next. It helps us to prepare for the new life we celebrate in December.

December: Patience

This is when the countdown officially begins for many students and teachers waiting for Christmas break to come. We all become antsy and have difficulty focusing on what we're supposed to. Student work tends to be sloppy, late, and incorrect. It's as if they don't care anymore. As teachers we wrestle with those same issues. It's sad that schools forget this beautiful season in the church. The rest we long for won't come with two weeks off. It comes only through the birth of our Lord Jesus Christ.

Advent is a time of waiting, conversion, and hope. We wait in the memory of the first coming of the Lord in mortal flesh. We also wait for His final, glorious coming as Lord and Judge. We pray for the conversion of all those who don't believe, quoting the prophets, especially John the Baptist. We have hope of the salvation already accomplished by Christ and in the fullness and maturity of our faith so that "we shall become like Him for we shall see Him as He really is" (1 John 3:2).

If you need a concrete way to focus on the coming of Jesus, use an Advent wreath. It's a respected European tradition to celebrate the Lord's birth and make hearts truly ready to receive Him. The symbolism of the wreath and its candles is stunning. The candles represent the coming of Light into the world. The circle of evergreen in which the candles are placed represents everlasting life. The four weeks before Christmas stir hearts in joyful anticipation of the Lord's coming. It's a much more satisfying and peaceful anticipation than Christmas break.

January: To Begin Again

New semester—clean slate! Why are you tired even before you begin at this time? Part of the reason is those two coveted weeks didn't accomplish what you'd hoped. Rest was replaced with the busyness of the season, and now you need a vacation from your vacation. Students aren't happy to be back, and their moans and groans make that quite clear. As you read down the list of names in your grade book, you now know your students well enough that each name conjures up an individual's character, behavior, and gifts and talents. To students your own name also invokes what they know and expect of you.

A name is a powerful thing. This month, ponder the name of Jesus, the name above every other name.

> *For this reason God also highly exalted Him and gave*
> *Him the name that is above every name, so that at the*
> *name of Jesus every knee should bow—of those who are*
> *in heaven and on earth and under the earth—and every*
> *tongue should confess that Jesus Christ is Lord, to the*
> *glory of God the Father. (Phil. 2:9–11)*

Names represent reputations. But it is not your reputation at stake. Consider how your thoughts, actions, and attitudes reflect on the name of Jesus. All that you do, you do to the glory of God. Focus now on how what you do as a Christian teacher displays the attributes associated with the name of Jesus. Do all things in His name.

February: Filling in Gaps, Mending Cracks

February is a short, yet difficult month. You work very hard on what now seems mundane. You follow an established routine almost on autopilot. Student gaps in learning are evident at this point, and you realize you may have to make changes to fill those gaps. You don't seem to have the energy to do more than the routine and find it difficult to come up with new ways to serve students. Your willingness to serve begins to lag, and your efforts may be halfhearted. You need a spiritual shot in the arm, a reminder of why you went into teaching in the first place.

During February, the church celebrates the presentation of the Lord at the temple. Although an expected ritual among the Jews of that time, it was also the outward act of presenting Jesus for humble service to God. Mary and Joseph presented Jesus at the temple as an act of sacrificial love. They expressed their obedience to the Mosaic Law through a ritual offering. It was a precursor to the offering Christ made at the cross, one of sacrificial love. It wasn't a payback; rather, it was a pure expression of love.

Meditate on Jesus' example by giving yourself without counting the cost or measuring the benefits. Choose to meet the needs of students. Do it sacrificially, out of charity and out of humble service to the Lord.

March: Weeding and Feeding

With the approach of spring comes the promise of new life and the fullness of a blossoming garden. The soil is prepared, planted, and watered. But weeds pop up, attempting to choke out your best efforts, and you have to remember to feed the still growing seedlings. Students, like a growing garden, still need a gardener even when the gardener is weary of tending.

Maybe you've let some of them fall through the cracks. Maybe their individual needs just seem too much to handle. Maybe desperate longing for the upcoming spring break clouds your desire to take care of those in your charge. It's understandable, but you can't stay that way.

At this point you must prepare your heart and mind for the greatest love offering of all time. Christ died while you were still a sinner. He paid the ultimate price for salvation when sinners were least deserving. Out of a grateful heart you can love your students in that same way and tend to their needs whether you feel like it or not, whether you think they deserve it or not.

Lent is characterized by penitence. Look for ways to repent of worldly attitudes and behaviors in order to fully comprehend why Jesus had to come and give Himself up for your sake. Search your heart and ask God to reveal to you anything you've said, thought, or done that might not have met the needs of a child in your care. Everyone's found lacking and falls short. If you're tired of dealing with a particular student's weakness, work harder to help her. If you're avoiding a particular parent, turn and meet him. If you've been defensive when your actions are questioned, submit and look for ways to improve. You aren't perfect. The sooner you acknowledge that and seek ways to reconcile and renew relationships, the sooner you'll experience the peace God promises.

April: Season of Renewal

This is usually a month of testing. You spend the last moments preparing and then spend the rest of the time actually testing. It's tedious and time-consuming. In fact, it's all-consuming! Your thoughts revolve around what you must do and when. You have procedures to follow and clocks to watch. Sadly, this has become the climax of the school year, the time everything leads to.

No wonder Easter is now just another Sunday. Yes, you may attend services and have a family feast, but attention to the climax of the church year falls flat. It has turned into one more thing on the to-do list. If you're to truly experience God's promised rest, meditate on the fullness of the gospel—Christ has died, Christ is risen, and Christ will come again! Go from the soberness of sin to the saving grace of Christ's death and resurrection. The world you touch can know through you the liberating, redeeming, and eternal truth of the gospel.

Even while you test students, they will know from your countenance and attitude that something is coming—something wonderful! While other teachers complain about the disruption of their schedules and their lack of teaching time, focus on the Lord's passion and the salvation gained because of it. Display the glory of the Lord at this time so others may ask about the peace you feel in the middle of their storm.

May: Spring Harvest

Testing is over, and now you do everything in your power to finish units and tie up loose ends. Grades must be turned in, award ceremonies are held, and yearbooks distributed. Final efforts are made to make sure students are equipped for the year to come. It's a busy time, and you feel the time is short and the tasks are many.

Even though Easter Sunday is over, the church calendar is still within the Easter season. It's not an end but a beginning. The church celebrates Pentecost, fifty days after Easter, the day on which the Holy Spirit descended on the apostles in the form of tongues of fire. The Holy Spirit gave the apostles the gifts they needed in order to undertake the evangelization of the world. They were equipped and then sent out to do God's work.

As you enter the final grades for your students, be sure you have properly equipped them to go forth with their lives. Focus first on your own equipping, and then focus on your students. The gifts of the Spirit enable you to do the work God created for you to His glory. Consider your gifts and renew your commitment to use them for God's glory.

June: Summer Solstice

The lazy, hazy days of summer arrive. Some teachers work a second job in the summer to make ends meet. Some teach summer school. Others look for ways to escape the heat and find restful vacation spots. Still others reconnect with much loved but often delayed activities and people they didn't have a chance to enjoy during the school year. And for some the to-do list is so long that rest is nowhere to be found. The promise of the next ten weeks brings with it a challenge. You try to accomplish reconnection, rest, and restoration all at the same time. How do you stay focused on important things when all you really want to do is escape?

June is the month the church contemplates the mystery of the Holy Trinity. This mystery doesn't fit easily into a specific calendar sequence, so you must exercise your faith to understand the concept. You may have difficulties multitasking, and because of human limitations, that's no surprise. But the Trinity accomplishes all in complete harmony and during the creation of the world still made time to rest.

The goal as you contemplate the Holy Trinity is not to unravel the mystery, but to immerse yourself in it and revel in its complex simplicity. St. Patrick attempted to illustrate the Trinity by using a three-leaf shamrock. Three in one and one in three. That's what Patrick saw in it—the beautiful mystery of the Father, the Son, and the Holy Spirit.

The mysteries of your faith bring peace, not anxiety or rest-lessness. Rest in the harmony of the Holy Trinity.

July: Careful Preparation

It's the middle of July, and now I count how many weeks until the first day of school. Another countdown. Sometimes I spend so much time looking toward what's to come that I miss seeing what's around today. Any preparations for the coming school year are not for myself. They're for the new children in my charge.

I wonder who will be on my roster this year. I wonder who will be my joy, who will drive me crazy, and who will make me laugh. Soberly I wonder whom I might not reach, whose struggles will fluster me, and whose home life will unnerve me. There are coming discoveries in a few weeks—good and bad.

God is never surprised by what He discovers about us. He is not caught off guard, unaware, or lacking. He loves us—all of us. He loves our students, even those who don't measure up, whose parents are antagonistic, and whose neediness make us want to run the other way. Take this time to rediscover in God how to love the unlovable and help the helpless. Prepare your heart for the coming year by lining it first with God's uncondi-tional and sacrificial love.

Don't focus on the days, months, and seasons without focusing on Christ. All that you focus on should point to Christ. Use the opportunities to refocus your view away from the world and onto Jesus' saving grace.

Days turn into weeks and weeks into months until you complete the year. You can go through it with your to-do list, or you can refocus your view on the love and words of Christ. Just as Martha and Mary differed in their approach to using time in Jesus' company, remember that Jesus said, "Mary has made the right choice, and it will not be taken away from her" (Luke 10:42). There are things you must do in life—people to serve, tasks to complete—but you can make the right choice and find ways to sit at His feet and contemplate His life and words. That's the place of rest!

Rest Stops
Take time each day to listen to your favorite music. Half an hour of music has been shown to produce the same effects of ten milligrams of Valium.[4]

Rest Reminders
For the Lord GOD, the Holy One of Israel, has said:
"You will be delivering by returning and resting;
your strength will lie in quiet confidence.
But you are not willing."
ISAIAH 30:15

My body, soul and spirit thus redeemed,
Sanctified and healed I give, O Lord, to Thee,
A consecrated offering, Thine evermore to be.

That all my powers with all their might
In thy sole glory may unite.
HENRY WILSON

Journal Prompt

At whatever point in the school year you read this,
stop, look, and listen. Stop your focus on the school calendar.
Look around at what God has accomplished during this time.
Listen for His voice and turn to follow it.

Chapter Eleven

The Test of Rest

You rejoice in this, though now for a short time you have
had to be distressed by various trials so that the genuineness
of your faith—more valuable than gold, which perishes
though refined by fire—may result in praise, glory, and
honor at the revelation of Jesus Christ.
1 PETER 1:6–7

I WAS COMPLETELY PREPARED, or so I thought. There
were going to be three days of testing in the week, so I checked
and double-checked my testing materials to make sure I had
everyone's booklets and response forms. Yes, all accounted for.

We spent weeks preparing for this testing session. The kids
knew how to behave and how to fill out the student information
portion and knew to bring a book to read if they finished early.
Parents stocked our teachers lounge with nutritious snacks for
the breaks, and everyone was reminded to have a good night's
sleep and a good breakfast on testing days. We were ready.

I knew what to do if something went wrong—and something always went wrong. The important thing was not to stop
the test. I had to deal with whatever happened in such a way as
not to invalidate the testing procedure. And if it was something
I didn't know how to handle, I had a chain of command to follow to get the situation under control.

Did you ever get all your ducks in a row only to find out that what you really needed were chickens? During that carefully prepared testing session, I discovered partway into it that my students were taking the wrong form of the test! I gave them form B when they were supposed to take form G. Somehow, no amount of attention to detail prevented this disaster. It caused quite a bit of inconvenience, to say the least.

Trials and tribulation, frustrations and failure come with teaching. After all, we're dealing with an imperfect product— human beings. Sometimes trouble comes from our own lacking, and other times it's because of someone else's deficiency. Either way, trouble comes and makes many teachers turn tail and run.

Wherever teachers gather they compare notes. The laundry list of complaints is growing out of control. Teachers are leaving the field like an army in full retreat. States can't fill positions fast enough. The North Carolina Professional Practices Commission, a group that monitors precollegiate teaching in the state, explains that "conditions teachers face in North Carolina are driving them out of the profession at a rate so high that the very foundations of public education in the state are threatened."[5] North Carolina is not alone. This is an international issue, not confined to teachers in the United States.

Teachers in New York leave in droves. More than eleven thousand of New York City's eighty thousand public school teachers stop teaching.[6] Retirement accounts for some of these, but a majority of these teachers are just fed up. They cite poor administrative support, lack of involvement in school decision making, and a poorly disciplined student body as their main reasons.

BBC News Online reports that "more than half of England's teachers expect to leave the profession within a decade because of stress, bureaucracy and heavy workloads."[7] Problems in relationships with colleagues are also commonly cited as sources of stress. Being a good teacher takes an emotional toll on a person. According to Vicky Condalary, a veteran teacher in Louisiana, "You reach the point where you're just watching the clock, trying to get through the day, whether the students are learning or not."[8] The losers are primarily the students. They deserve teachers who are not burned out or out of touch as they anesthetize themselves from the onslaught of emotionally crippling trials and troubles of teaching.

Is there hope? Can we really find rest and renewal amid what threatens to destroy us? King David asked the same question. I include Psalm 27 in its entirety to give you a chance to recognize your own trouble, fears, and the source of your salvation, protection, and peace.

> *The LORD is my light and my salvation—*
> *whom should I fear?*
> *The LORD is the stronghold of my life—*
> *of whom should I be afraid?*
> *When evildoers came against me to devour my flesh,*
> *my foes and my enemies stumbled and fell.*
> *Though an army deploy against me,*
> *my heart is not afraid;*
> *though war break out against me,*
> *still I am confident.*
> *I have asked one thing from the LORD; it is what I desire:*
> *to dwell in the house of the LORD all the days of my life,*
> *gazing on the beauty of the LORD*
> *and seeking Him in His temple.*
> *For He will conceal me in His shelter in the day of adversity;*
> *He will hide me under the cover of His tent;*
> *He will set me high on a rock.*
> *Then my head will be high above my enemies around me;*
> *I will offer sacrifices in His tent with shouts of joy.*

I will sing and make music to the LORD.
LORD, hear my voice when I call;
be gracious to me and answer me.
In Your behalf my heart says, "Seek My face."
LORD, I will seek Your face.
Do not hide Your face from me;
do not turn Your servant away in anger.
You have been my help;
do not leave me or abandon me,
God of my salvation.
Even if my father and mother abandon me,
the LORD cares for me.
Because of my adversaries,
show me Your way, LORD,
and lead me on a level path.
Do not give me over to the will of my foes,
for false witnesses rise up against me, breathing violence.
I am certain that I will see the LORD's goodness
in the land of the living.
Wait for the LORD;
be courageous and let your heart be strong.
Wait for the LORD.

The Enemy keeps track of how many good teachers he's driven away from the classroom because of trials and troubles. Don't misunderstand me—trials will come even if you're steadfast in the Lord. But the Enemy will not waste an opportunity to shake your belief that you're where you belong. Even Christian teachers are shaken to the core by some of what goes on in our schools. You may fall into the trap of looking for earthly ways to get out of this trouble. What students, parents, colleagues, and administrators meant for evil, God meant for good (Gen. 50:20). How can you use what's thrown at you for your good and God's glory?

Trials Mature Our Faith

> *Consider it a great joy, my brothers, whenever you experience various trials, knowing that the testing of your faith produces endurance. But endurance must do its complete work, so that you may be mature and complete, lacking nothing. (James 1:2–4)*

I left and returned to teaching three times. I think the third time is the charm! The first seven years I taught, everything was new to me. Everything that happened took me by surprise. The second time I taught, I thought I knew it all and found out I knew some things, but plenty of new challenges threw me for a loop. Now the third time around, I know many things I didn't know before, such as no matter what my principal throws at me, my God is in control. I know I can love the most unlovable students if I allow God to love them through me. I know compassion will take me far. I know appreciation for others' talents will put my mind at ease in difficult situations. I know these things because God taught them to me through trials the first two times. And I'm sure I still have a lot to learn, so I'm sure the third time will offer me many more opportunities to learn and mature.

Trials have a purpose. They don't come by accident, nor should we be taken by surprise. Jesus told us they would come. He did not want us ignorant. The key is to recognize them for what they are quickly so we don't wallow in despair and miss the blessing that's sure to follow.

Trials Prove Our Faith

> *Blessed is a man who endures trials, because when he passes the test he will receive the crown of life that He has promised to those who love Him. (James 1:12)*

When I taught literature to middle school students, I trained them in the Socratic questioning method, which says that a student may express an opinion as long as he provides evidence for it. When asked a "why" question, he must provide an answer and be able to refer back to the reading selection and supply evidence from the text. We had quite a few discussions that ran overtime as students debated their evidence. It was quite exciting!

Remember the discussions Satan had with God about Job (Job 8–11). They each had an opinion.

God: Have you considered my servant Job? No one else on earth is like him, a man of perfect integrity, who fears God and turns away from evil.

Satan: You have blessed the work of his hands, and his possessions are spread out in the land. But stretch out Your hand and strike everything he owns, and he will surely curse You to Your face.

The rest of the story is a matter of evidence. In the end God's evidence of Job's character prevailed. Job's faith withstood his trials and was proven.

The test is upon you. The trials of the unresponsive student, the unruly parent, noncommensurate salaries, the undermining colleague, or the unresponsive administrator all look to prove your faith. Your response is the evidence. What will that evidence prove about you?

Caution

No one undergoing a trial should say, "I am being tempted by God." For God is not tempted by evil, and He Himself doesn't tempt anyone. But each person is tempted when he is drawn away and enticed by his own evil desires. Then

after desire has conceived, it gives birth to sin, and when sin
is fully grown, it gives birth to death. (James 1:13–15)

Many teach using a sequence. One thing naturally leads to another. Not only is that helpful as you plan to teach a particular subject, but it also helps pinpoint where you or students might have gone wrong if they fail. Usually the fault lies in the beginning when the concept is first taught. If a student doesn't grasp the concept at first, your response can lead her to one of two places—success or failure. If you give in to the belief that you don't have time to address her learning gap, it becomes a much bigger hole and a much bigger problem to solve. If you ignore the problem at this point, it's like trying to drive around a sinkhole in the road, growing right before your eyes.

How you first respond to the trial can indicate which sequence you end up following—one that leads to life or one that leads to death. You can deny the trial, run away from it, fight it, or face it with full confidence that God is with you. Sometimes you may allow fear to dictate which path you take. You give in to the fear and turn away from the trial in panic. The more you avoid trials, the less you'll grow. The only way to really grow in Christ is to go through trials with Him at your side.

I will be with you when you pass through the waters,
and when you pass through the rivers,
they will not overwhelm you.
You will not be scorched when you walk through the fire,
and the flame will not burn you. (Isa. 43:2)

When you pass through the waters. *When* you pass through the rivers. *When* you walk through the fire. The operative word here is *when*. As you read this, your life may be going smoothly. But things will go wrong—they always do. And when they do, when you feel the water slipping over your head, when you feel powerless against the rapids of the rushing river, or when you feel the hairs on your arms begin to scorch because of the heat, remember God is with you. He's not somewhere far away, looking down and shaking His head in dismay. He's right there in the thick of it with you. When your principal scolds you in front of the entire faculty. When a parent undermines your authority. When a student takes a swing at you during hall duty. When your own children seem out of control, or your spouse isn't satisfied with how much time you spend with him or her. God is with you—*through* the waters, *through* the rivers, and *through* the fire. On that you can rely. In that you can finally rest.

Rest Stops

Teachers drink too much coffee and too many soft drinks. Caffeine is the second most common stimulant. You may not realize how it adds up over the course of a school day. Excessive amounts of caffeine can cause restlessness, insomnia, heart irregularities, and even panic attacks. Substitute high-protein snacks like cheese, nuts, or seeds instead of heading to the lounge for another cup of joe.

Rest Reminders

You rejoice in this, though now for a short time you have had to be distressed by various trials so that the genuineness of your faith—more valuable than gold, which perishes though refined by fire—may result in praise, glory, and honor at the revelation of Jesus Christ.

1 PETER 1:6–7

Crosses are Ladders to Heaven.

THOMAS FULLER

Journal Prompt

Are you facing a trial as an educator? What is your usual response? What have you learned in this chapter to help you go *through* the trial?

Chapter Twelve

The Yearbook of Rest

Therefore, as a fellow elder and witness to the sufferings
of the Messiah, and also a participant in the glory about to
be revealed, I exhort the elders among you: shepherd God's
flock among you, not overseeing out of compulsion but
freely, according to God's will; not for the money but
eagerly; not lording it over those entrusted to you,
but being examples to the flock.
1 PETER 5:1–3
(emphasis added)

FINDING REST IS something every person on this planet tries
to do. Each situation, each occupation, has its own unique challenges, frustrations, and disappointments that make rest difficult to find if you don't know where to look. Suggestions usually
are more readily accepted from someone who really knows what
your life is like. The best source of ideas about how to find rest
is other teachers.

We can be examples to one another for how to find rest in
healthy, productive, and God-honoring ways. We can be rest
mentors! We mentor other teachers not for an additional stipend
to our pay but with enthusiasm for the greater glory of God.

The foundation of real rest comes only by the Father, Son,
and Holy Spirit, but some ideas can refresh and renew your

body, mind, and spirit. The teachers on the following pages share how they find rest as educators. As you gain a glimpse into their lives, I hope you will be encouraged on your quest toward rest.

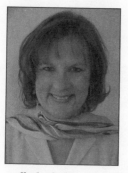

Prayerwalking

By Janet Holm McHenry

Paradoxically, the best hour of rest I have each day is the hour after I wake up each morning. In five fast minutes, I throw on fleece layers and my walking shoes, grab my walking poles, and head out onto the streets of my small community in the California Sierra. There I walk the half mile of Main Street under the streetlights—getting great exercise and even greater time with God, praying for the people in Loyalton.

I started prayerwalking more than six years ago when I hit a crisis point. I was tired all the time. I was huffing and puffing just climbing the stairs in our home. I couldn't fall asleep without painkillers—my joints ached so much. The worst moment was when I stepped out our back door one day and found myself in a crumpled heap because my knee had given way.

I determined then and there that I would get up a little earlier the next morning and start walking. As a busy high school English teacher and mom to four kids, I also find I must multitask through my days, so I also decided to use the time to pray. While my prayers were very "I-centered" when I began, that all changed one morning when I saw a young daddy drop off his baby girl at a day-care center before six in the morning. When she said, "Bye, Daddy," I knew God wanted me to begin praying for the needs in my little town. Soon my prayer hour was flying by as I prayed for the business owners and neighbors around me. A short time later, I asked a teacher friend to join me one day a week, and we now prayerwalk around the four schools in our town, praying for each teacher by name and for larger school issues.

I've experienced dramatic changes in my life because of prayerwalking. Depression and fears that plagued me for years evaporated, my aches and pains vanished, and I've lost two dress sizes. It's kind of crazy, but even though I get a little less sleep than I used to, I feel more rested at the end of a day. Some might think prayerwalking isn't a restful activity, but I find that when I hand over my burdens to God each day, my load is much lighter as I head back to my house, to my workday, to my classroom, and even to the teachers' room!

Janet Holm McHenry teaches high school English, journalism, and creative writing at Loyalton High School in Loyalton, California, where she also is adviser for the senior class, California Scholarship Federation, Grizzly Writers' Society, and the school newspaper. She loves scoring basketball games and writing. You can read about her book *Prayer Changes Teens: How to Parent from Your Knees* at www.dailyprayerwalking.com.

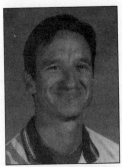

A Teacher's Rest

By Stephan Melancon

As a teacher I find rest without looking for it. Someone very important to me said, "For whoever wants to save his life will lose it, but whoever loses his life because of Me will find it" (Matt. 16:25). I lose my life for my students. It isn't nearly as lofty or holy as it sounds. I simply attempt to put their needs before my own. I don't try to escape from them. When I look for rest specifically as a respite from my work, I almost never feel rested. Teaching for me is essentially mission work. I've been called to serve a group of people whose needs are immediate and very different from my own. Rest from mission work involves doing something different from day-to-day demands, but it still involves doing. To re-create myself, I do things for others that, in the process, strengthen my own body, mind, and soul.

Coaching benefits me as much as it does my players. I run every mile my student athletes run. They know I expect no more of them than I'm willing to give myself. Coaching allows me to make connections with my students on a very different level than in the classroom. We run, laugh, sweat, ache, and celebrate together. At night, I sleep. I sleep very well.

I also feel rested when my mind is clear, and my mind is clearer, sharper, when it's fully engaged. When I talk with my students about topics we have beaten to death, such as grades, homework, teachers, or rules, I often grow weary. But I literally never tire; in fact I'm invigorated when we talk about subjects of more substance. I make myself available to the young people in my life in and out of school. I'm refreshed by the wit and even wisdom of their "new" minds. They make me think. When I'm sought out, and especially when I'm challenged or called on to defend an apparently outdated position, I'm honored. I'm stimulated. I'm clear-minded.

Worry clouds my mind and causes tension. When I worry, I feel it in my neck. For those students for whom I worry most, I pray. Actually, I try to pray for the ones who appear to be doing just fine as well. I try to see my students as resilient creatures who can and will bounce back from their seemingly overwhelming obstacles. I can see them this way only through the eyes of faith. Faith leads to hope. Hope and worry are incompatible.

When I pray for my students, I have hope for them. I have faith that they can become what they were created to be. Then I don't have to worry. Then I can relax. Then I can rest.

Stephan Melancon serves as a resource specialist, or teacher of students with special needs, at a small, rural high school in northern California's Sierra Valley. He is the husband of Betsy Melancon, the high school's library aide, who also serves the area as a midwife. Stephan is the proud father of five, including David Christian, a ten-year-old; three teenage girls, Theresa Jayne, Nicole Antoinette, and Selina Rae; and an eighteen-year-old Sean Francis. Stephan and his family are devout Roman Catholics. Stephan has a bachelor of science degree in special education from the University of Nevada, Las Vegas, with graduate work in early childhood education and reading.

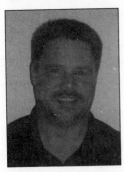

Vanishing

By Tony Horning

A number of surveys can offer an estimate of the number of expectations, requests, and demands placed on or generated by an educator during an average school day. I've experienced the heavy weight of those expectations as a classroom teacher, college professor, and school administrator. Anyone who has had a class or school under his leadership understands how crushing those expectations can be. And beyond the stressful occurrences that can steal hours and even days is the sneaky, glacial buildup of apparently invisible expectations within a busy day. Solomon stated, "the little foxes that ruin the vineyards" (Song of Sol. 2:15a), and those little foxes come in a seemingly unrelenting current against which we struggle regularly, even to the point of accepting the struggle as typical and perhaps, God forbid, *normal*.

The need for me to vanish surfaced when I became an administrator. Never before had I come to a place inside myself where I actually wanted to separate myself from everyone. I tried different remedies like TV and quiet time, but I always seemed to return to my duties tired and sometimes bitter about my plight. It was by surprise that I discovered fleeing from people wasn't what I needed, but rather moving among them without fear of ending my journey with a to-do list a mile long, which can happen when I simply walk down my school's hallways. This allowed me to nurture my appreciation for people instead of allowing my own issues to turn the people I have been called to love and serve into my enemies.

When I vanish, I must do it alone. I shouldn't take anyone with me. This applies to the people I enjoy because many times with these people I find myself replaying the less than positive aspects of my life; after all, that's what friends are for. No, when I vanish I get in my car and go to a place where I've never been and then walk around and take in the community, shops, and the peace of communing with the Lord. Vanishing allows me to momentarily escape the ever-present crush of expectations. Vanishing is the process of *coming apart* in order to keep from coming apart, but it is only when I choose to take Christ's yoke on myself, rather than everyone else's yoke, that I find true rest.

Tony Horning is a career educator who has experienced classroom teaching at the elementary, junior college, and college levels. His administrative experiences encompass both public and private schools. Currently, he is the founding director of ArtSpace Charter School near Asheville, North Carolina. He lives in Black Mountain, North Carolina, with his wife, Jane, and their children, Jacob and Elizabeth.

A Change of Pace

By Harvey Rachlin

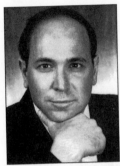

After years of writing books full time, I felt I was in a major rut and needed something to get me out of my basement office and into the world. When I began my writing career, I taught for a short while to provide income, but I dreamed of giving it up so I could devote myself to pouring my thoughts onto paper and seeing them appear in print. Writing books became an obsession; teaching was OK, but even part time, it seemed like a distraction. After I nailed down a few book contracts, I was financially able to quit, and I did.

Several books later, though, I began to feel out of touch and realized I needed to spend more time interacting with people to keep my writing fresh. I thought about teaching again, and it seemed like the perfect solution—limited hours yet mentally challenging. I was fortunate enough to be hired by Manhattanville College in Purchase, New York, in 1996, and I continue teaching there today with the title of adjunct professor.

While at first I considered teaching as no more than a rut-breaker, I now find with each new semester I love it more. It takes my mind off the "business" of writing—the anxiety of waiting for a phone call from an editor or agent, the disappointment of a rejection—and puts me in a good mood. Most of all, I've become hooked on teaching because of the respect I get from my students. They call me professor, look at me a little starry-eyed, and address me with a degree of reverence. What a contrast to the attitudes of editors and family members—even though by this time I have a dozen books and a TV show to my credit!

As a writer/teacher I lead a double life: a few days a week I am a bestubbled, jeans-and-T-shirt-clad, anxiety-ridden author; and the other days I am a clean-shaven, elegantly dressed, confident academic. By the time I get into the classroom, the metamorphosis from sullen, withdrawn writer to dynamic, gregarious professor stuns even me.

At the end of my teaching day I get into my car, still on a high from my day in front of my students. At some point during the ride home, I remember I'm waiting to hear from an editor or agent on a new book proposal, and maybe today will be the day I get the news. But I tell myself that even if it doesn't turn out the way I'd hoped, I won't be upset. Teaching has taught me that writing isn't the most important thing in the world.

Harvey Rachlin is the author of twelve books, including, most recently, *Lucy's Bones, Sacred Stones, and Einstein's Brain* and *Jumbo's Hide, Elvis's Ride, and the Tooth of Buddha*, which were adapted for the History Channel's "History's Lost and Found" series. He's a winner of the ASCAP-Deems Taylor Award for excellence in music journalism and has written for numerous magazines and newspapers and appeared on hundreds of radio and TV shows. He is currently writing *Cloaks, Daggers, and Da Vincis* for Penguin Books.

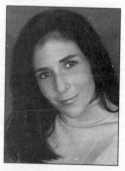

A Little R & R

By Kelly A. Hammer

Beep! Beep! Beep! The alarm sounds early at my house. After about a seven-hour sleep, the sound reminds me of a new day, a new beginning, a chance to renew my spirit. As I continue through the day, helping and caring for others, I realize none of my efforts would be sincere if I hadn't first nourished my own soul. All it takes for me is a little "R & R," my run and the rosary!

Being a mom of two small children, a preschool teacher, and a family nutritionist, I find little time to devote to myself. When the alarm sounds, I head out for my three-mile run and pray while doing so. Whether I finger each of the fifty glass beads, strung together on a chain, to keep track of my prayers or I mentally count them, it automatically cancels out my worries and focuses my prayers. Praying is a good distraction from the little worries I make so big. Like making sure my son doesn't forget his lunch or brushing my daughter's hair! More importantly, the prayers are a reminder of what truly matters in this life. I pray each day for a kind heart and a gentle touch with a focus to fill others with the same.

The constant changes and chaos of my day start early. Therefore, praying during my run seems to be the only constant I have. As it should be, my time with God above all things is paramount. What better way to start a day than to refocus on God's true and constant love. This time lasts only about thirty minutes each morning, but without it, the day would be much more treacherous.

The precious children I care for at the preschool, the families in need I counsel, and most importantly my own family all deserve the best I can give them each day. My gift to others is only as good as I am to myself and to God. Like a deep well, it must first be filled with water before it's able to provide to others who are thirsty. So, too, must I first fill myself with the spirit of love to touch the people in my life honestly and lovingly.

Kelly A. Hammer teaches preschool at Cullowhee Kids at Cullowhee United Methodist Church in Sylva, North Carolina, where she is also founder and owner of Hammer Nutrition and works as a family health consultant. She also teaches fourth-grade catechism classes at St. Mary's Catholic Church and is a busy mom of two young children. Kelly has written for Focus on the Family and has her own Web site, www.brainfoods.biz, which provides information about how nutrition affects the brain and personal success in life.

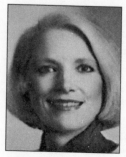

Doughnut Shop Daily Date

By Bonnie Afman Emmorey

Here I was, feeling chained to the home instead of the school. I had chosen to be a full-time mom for a few years instead of a teacher, but I was still married to a full-time teacher. With two boys under the age of four, I was as close to being a crazy woman as possible without actually going over the edge. Teaching was *easy* compared to what *I* was doing! I longed for the time when my husband arrived home and I could have an adult conversation. Unfortunately, he was longing for peace and quiet.

After being with kids all day, he needed to relax and unwind. But how could anyone relax when there were still papers to grade and lessons to plan? It was impossible for him to suddenly jump into family life at 4:00 p.m., especially when he was still being controlled by school demands. We were facing a dilemma. I needed a husband who could carry on an adult conversation and make me feel like a *normal adult,* and our children needed a daddy to play with and enjoy.

It was by sheer chance that the answer presented itself. One afternoon, Ron was running behind schedule at school and knew I would worry if he didn't make it home at the usual time. He called and suggested I pack up the boys and meet him at the local doughnut shop halfway between school and home. We sat in a booth and had coffee while reading the paper. Within a half hour or so, we were both totally relaxed and ready to talk. It was amazing how conversation flowed. Our sons had entertained themselves and played quietly, and Ron found he was able to leave school behind. I was out in the real world with people who could actually talk as adults. It was almost as good as the teachers' lounge!

As we evaluated what had happened, we discovered something amazing. When Ron would come straight home from school, he brought school with him. Unfortunately, he couldn't share it with *me*. But by meeting at a location away from school and away from home, we were both able to unwind and prepare for the rest of the day, the family portion of the day. It was like a minivacation for both of us every day. We started having a daily date at the doughnut shop.

There was only one small glitch in our new system. We soon discovered he was so adept at leaving school at the shop, he was no longer able to get any message home to me. No problem. He just had the school call directly! It worked!

While Bonnie Afman Emmorey is not currently working in a traditional classroom, she's using her skills through Speak Up with Confidence Seminars, teaching communication skills from a Christian perspective. She is also a speaker consultant with Speak Up Speaker Services. Visit www.speakupspeaker services.com to learn more. Bonnie is currently involved in launching the new nonprofit organization Speak Up for Hope, with the goal of connecting churches with prisons and assisting chaplains in meeting the needs of prisoners and their families. For additional information, go to www.speakupforhope.com. Her husband, Ron, is a public school teacher in Gaylord, Michigan, and they have two sons. Bonnie says, "Living with three men has taught me the most!"

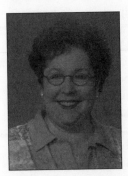

Rest and Renewal
By Cathy Gallagher

A year ago I discovered a truth about work, play, and renewal I didn't know I needed to learn.

For some people, work and play are separate entities—one begins where the other leaves off. Work provides income to pay bills and for fun activities that renew the spirit. For me, however, work *is* play—the two merge in a career position that makes my heart sing by allowing me to use skills and talents I most enjoy using in ways I most enjoy applying them.

The past two years, however, have been different. After an unprecedented loss of three jobs in eighteen months, the last shortly after 9/11, I accepted a job at Michigan's unemployment office. Because this job pays 50 percent less than I've ever earned and doesn't make my heart sing, I often felt mentally, emotionally, and spiritually drained.

As I reached out to God for help during prayer a year ago, I felt an inner prompting to read Bible verses about renewing the mind. As I read them, I realized for the first time in my thirty-year career, rest and renewal don't flow into me naturally from a job that blends my heart's desires, skills, and talents. Rather, rest and renewal will flow into me every day if I apply the Bible's principles about renewing my mind.

I stopped focusing on what this job isn't. I became thankful for what the job offers: an honorable source of income, wonderful health benefits, and the opportunity to learn new skills while working with colleagues I otherwise never would have met. I stopped looking at the day with drudgery as I awoke in the morning. I started praying that God would help me see and respond to the countless daily opportunities to make a difference in people's lives.

As my outlook became more positive, my exhaustion lifted. I had the energy to pursue volunteer opportunities through my church, to submit articles for publication, and to teach as an adjunct faculty member at local colleges and universities, which do make my heart sing.

Today, I know it's not a particular job that makes my heart sing, my attitude does: My heart can sing no matter what circumstances I face as long as I apply to my life the Bible's advice about renewing my mind.

Cathy Gallagher received her teaching certificate and bachelor of arts degree from Adrian College, Adrian, Michigan, and her master of arts in education from Michigan State University. She has held a myriad of positions in the business world, including unemployment claims examiner, salesperson, marketing manager, customer service director, and assistant dean. She is an adjunct faculty member at a local college and university. More than twenty-five of her articles have been published, one in *Guideposts*. She has ghostwritten a book on business communications for an established author. Cathy speaks and writes from her life experiences. Her topics include "Enlisting God's Help in Career Transitions," "Release through God's Word," "The Power of a Transformed Life," and "Prayer." To receive information on scheduling Cathy as a speaker for an event, go to www.speakupspeakerservices.com or call 1-888-870-7719.

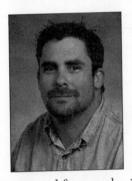

Take the Long Way Home

By Chad Guercia

Five years ago I switched professions from a high-stress, deadline-filled job to teaching high school. I soon realized I had it easy at my old job. I wasn't ready for the demands and attention from parents, students, and faculty.

The first month of teaching I returned from work with the weight of the world on my shoulders. I soon found out I had no choice but to bring my work home with me. The only aspect of teaching I felt I had control over was what type of work I was going to bring home. I had to make a change to keep my sanity along with my professionalism.

I made several changes that were key to my success over the past few years. First, I changed how I left the workplace. I took several minutes for myself at the end of the day to unwind before I started on my way home. To find peace in my mind and life, I would turn out the lights in the classroom, sit down at my desk, and cross my legs at the ankles and my arms across my chest. There I would sit and ponder my day and what I wanted to accomplish. This type of mental and physical meditation would enable me to relax and let go before I left for the day.

Second, I started taking the long way home. This enabled me to put my mind somewhere else before I walked into the house to greet my wife and precious little dogs. I didn't want to bring the rigors of the day with me to pass on to my wife. This way, when I walked through that door, I was ready for and able to complete the second half of my day.

Finally, I joined a golf league with some of my coworkers and friends. We would meet once a week to play nine holes and enjoy one another's time and camaraderie. I found that golfing was a great form of physical and mental exercise. For the past few years I have enjoyed trying to knock a tiny white ball around a grass pasture only to realize that the stress of the day was nothing compared to proving to myself that every other shot I attempted was not up to my standards. This rejuvenated me because I understood that no matter how good I think I am, I still have imperfections I need to work on. This is how my students feel from time to time. I get to remember this when I forget to see why some of my students and parents feel frustrated during the school year.

Chad Guercia is a high school earth/space science teacher at Palm Harbor University High School in Palm Harbor, Florida. He is also a certified Brain Gym instructor for Integrated Learning Corp. (E-mail: integratedlc@msn.com). Chad enjoys coaching soccer and participating at school athletic events. In his spare time he plays golf and coaches athletes through integrated instruction and kinesiology.

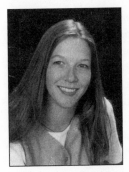

My Quiet Time

By Jennifer Bell

The alarm goes off at 6:00 a.m. Is it morning already? I drag myself out of bed, feed the dogs, shower, dress, and grab a quick breakfast. I then get breakfast for my son, get him dressed, say a quick good-bye to my husband, and head to day care.

At school, it's time to check my messages, get copies made for the day, and review my lesson plans. At 8:20 the bell rings. I take a deep breath. Here they come. As soon as the doors open, I hear a student yell, "What's for lunch?" Another student says, "Can I go to the bathroom?" The questions continue into the classroom: "What are we doing today?" "Can you help me with this?" "Do you know what I did last night?" and so on. Questions like this are hurled at me all day long. By 3:20 p.m., I'm ready for quiet time. Not yet.

I pick up my son and spend the late afternoon tending to his one-year-old needs: changing diapers, playing games, and eating a snack. Sometimes he takes a nap. I spend this time cleaning up, grading papers, or planning for the next day.

When he wakes up, it's time to start supper, play again, eat dinner, give him a bath, and put him down for the evening. At this point it's around 9:30. I still have a few odds and ends to finish up with the house or work. An hour or so later, I have my quiet time.

Although my day is very hectic and it seems I'm catering to everyone else's needs during the day, I wouldn't have it any other way. I find it quite relaxing to cross-stitch. It allows my mind to slow down and forget everything else that happened throughout the day. This hobby relaxes me more than anything else. I also enjoy reading. Reading helps my mind to escape from the reality of the daily hustle and bustle. Finally, I enjoy writing letters. Yes, you read that correctly. I enjoy writing letters. It gives me time to catch up with friends and family on a personal level. Once I finish my quiet time, I'm able to go to sleep with my mind at ease and let my body prepare itself for the next day.

Jennifer Bell taught fourth grade for five years. She now teaches fifth grade at Stetson Elementary in Colorado Springs. She is married and has one son.

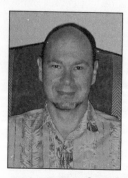

Morning Cup with God
By Jim Zabloski

I'm a self-admitted edu-holic. I live to learn and to teach others how to learn. Whether I do that through teaching or through writing, I've given my voice and my hands to the Lord for the education of others. I am called. I am driven. Finding rest in the midst of such self-motivation can be a difficult thing. Complicate that with the surrounding Miami skyline and traffic noise, and the reality of rest takes real effort.

Several years ago my wife (also a teacher) and I decided to sell our suburban home and move to "the country" for peace, quiet, and rest. Country is about as easy to find in Miami as snow in December. Our search took us to only eight pieces of property, and we found a fixer-upper in an area where the homes are on acre-plus lots. It's not exactly Wyoming, but we took it. It's only an eighth of a mile from a main road, but it's the last house on a dead-end street and bordering a canal.

Here I found my rest. I discovered that if I get up early enough, sit out on the patio long enough, sip several cups of coffee slowly while talking with my Father, I am rested. I listen to the buffo frogs serenade their last bit of evening song while I talk with God. The mockingbirds choose from a variety of songs until they find just the right one for the day while I commune with Him. Our beagle occasionally bays at the discovery of a long-lost scent from the evening past while God encourages me. While the city slowly awakens, God and I are just finishing up.

It wasn't always like this. For years while I taught elementary school, I jumped out of bed and headed off to the classroom prepared to deliver lesson plans but unprepared for spiritual warfare. That battle can be long and arduous, and too many days of that wore me out. I kept up the frenetic pace when I went into publishing and writing, more often than not putting in sixteen-hour days. Marriage. Kids. Mortgages. Nothing slowed me down, until I somehow awakened to the notion that this life is the temporary one, and the eternal one is getting closer. I suppose I never understood how important rest—true soul rest—is, until I reached my mid-forties.

It doesn't take an acre on a canal to do that. I'm certain I could've had my cup of java with God in the 'burbs as well. But there is something magical about the sounds and sights of morning, alone and quiet, that seems to bring rest when nothing else will.

Jim Zabloski taught sixth grade for six years, moved into the publishing field for a decade, and then returned to teach college for one year. He wrote *The 25 Most Common Problems in Business* and dozens of plays and sketches. He now is a part-time freelance writer working on three book projects. A full-time pastor in a large church in Fort Lauderdale, Florida, he oversees the adult education and small-group ministries.

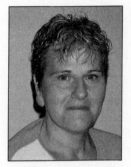

Addicted to Reading

By Linda Zabloski

"Today, class, we will read . . ." "Open your books to page 37 and begin reading . . ." "The novel we will be reading this year is . . ." These words are usually followed by various moans and groans. My heart breaks a little. Reading is my refuge, and I'm saddened that so many young people see it as a burden. Yes, you can rent the DVD and read the Cliffs Notes, but to me devouring a book is an opportunity to rest.

Teachers often joke that the three reasons they teach are June, July, and August. I would never go that far, but I will admit those are my prime reading months. During the school year I find it difficult to find time to read. Understand, though, I am an addicted reader. I just can't sit for a few minutes and read a chapter. I can read for hours at a time, often finishing books in two days. I have disciplined myself to save my reading adventures for the summer. I count it a wonderful, restful summer when I have been able to read books and sleep in.

Some summers I am on an author phase. I have read all of John Grisham's books in one summer. That very summer I visited my sister in Virginia and met Grisham in her country store. I am a Jerry Jenkins fan, and I'm frustrated at times that I have to wait so long for his next book. Mostly, I read mysteries and let my mind rest in the adventures of others.

I also try to do a reading project with my sons during the summer. Recently, we read through the book of Proverbs and chose a verse to share. We visit the library and come home with stacks of books. I want my children to love to read and find the joy in a good book.

I know some people would see reading as just another exercise for their brain and not restful at all, but for a book lover it's a way to escape and find time to let one's mind wander. I'm careful to choose books that are uplifting and God-honoring. I just finished two Francine Rivers books that actually had me weeping over God's love and goodness. I mentioned this to a friend at church, who also had read one of the books, and we relived the blessing of a good book.

As my summer ends, I know my marathon reading sessions are over. I'll still keep a few books on the nightstand and squeeze in a few moments before I sleep. I can't stop completely. I'm a compulsive reader, but I am renewed and ready to challenge my students: "Open your books to page 37."

Linda Zabloski is beginning her seventeenth year of teaching. She has taught elementary and high school classes. Her favorite age group is the notorious middle school. These students' enthusiasm and energy match her zest for life. She speaks at women's conferences, teaches Bible studies, and loves spending time with her husband and two sons.

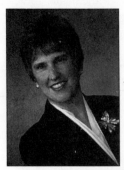

A Gardener's Rest

By Karen Allaman

I enjoy watching things grow! I am a gardener by birth, temperament, and habit. Spring, summer, and fall bring flower gardens, an herb garden, a corn garden, and a vegetable garden. I plant annuals, transplant bulbs, sow seeds, and split tubers.

I love it all—the preparing, the planting, and the harvesting. I feel such reward as I watch God make the flowers grow. I marvel at the bounty of the vegetable harvest He provides. Time flies as I quietly prune, weed, and transplant.

My senses are awakened in my garden. Stress and pressures fade away with each twist of my trowel. As the crocus, daffodils, tulips, lily of the valley, bleeding heart, dill, and tomatoes come to bud and blossom, the worries of last year's school year are forgotten, and hope buds and blooms again. I find myself renewed and revitalized.

My first gardening attempts failed miserably as I fussed and fumed about placement of just the right plant in just the right spot, worried about colors in the garden and the proper light, water, and soil. I obsessed about overwatering or underfertilizing. I purchased all kinds of gadgets, special fertilizers, and the latest trend in gardening. The joy I expected never came because I exhausted myself with trivial aspects of gardening that didn't make a bit of difference to the plants.

After a few years of fighting with my garden and trying to improve on nature's way of taking everything in its own season, I decided to go back to what brought me to the garden in the first place: love for the plants and flowers. As the plants grew, I began to observe the signs of overwatering or pests. It was in the quiet times of observation that I became aware of what the flowers truly needed to thrive. It was not through the gadgets, trends, or fads that I found the best results. It was in the consistent care of a watchful eye. It was then that the delight of gardening became apparent, and I have been hooked ever since.

A gardener's touch is a useful tool in my classroom, both for the gardener and the student. I love to watch plants and children grow!

Karen Allaman lives with her husband in a small town in western Pennsylvania. They have two grown children. Karen holds a master's degree in elementary education and is certified as a reading specialist. She is an avid gardener and storyteller. Karen enjoys speaking for Stonecroft Ministries, seminars, women's groups, Bible schools, and banquets.

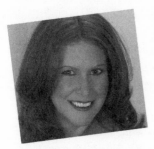

No Idle Hands

By Vicki Caruana

"What are you making?" the passenger next to me on the airplane asks.

"Is that a scarf?" a colleague asks in the teachers lounge.

"Is that knitting or crochet?" the mom on the playground wonders.

What I do to relax always attracts attention and elicits questions from those around me. To me, knitting is as peaceful as sleeping is to other people. When I'm stressed, fearful, or anxious I knit. In many years my knitting projects outnumbered anything else I did for that year—some years were more stressful than others.

I learned a long time ago it's good to keep my hands busy—hands busy when I'm riding in the car, hands busy when I'm waiting in the doctor's office, hands busy when I'm worried about something. My great aunt Flo taught me this when I was nine, the summer I scraped my knees so badly I had to sit out the whole summer. She taught me how to knit so I would have no idle hands and a heart at peace. It worked then, and it works for me now.

I've never made anything for myself. Every new baby among my family and friends has received a baby blanket. Every newlywed couple has received an afghan. I've made scarves, sweaters, ponchos, mittens, and footies for those who live where it's cold. At this point in my life, I've run out of things to make for my family, so now I send the works of my hands outward.

Every school year my students see my current knitting project nestled in a black bag next to my desk. It always intrigues them. Sometimes they ask for lessons. What a joy that is. Now when they ask whom I'm making something for, I tell them I knit for charity. I knit for orphaned children of Afghanistan. I knit for our troops in various parts of the world. I knit baby blankets for neonatal care units at area hospitals. This brings even more peace to my weary soul as I use a talent God has given me to meet physical needs of His people.

Teaching can be both mentally and spiritually exhausting. I use a lot of energy to come up with new ideas and new ways of helping children. I have to be creative. Knitting allows me to be creative with my hands—something my job often doesn't give me a chance to be.

Vicki Caruana has spent much of her career encouraging teachers through the written and spoken word. Her best-selling books include *Apples & Chalkdust: Inspiration and Encouragement for Teachers* and *When Teachers Pray.* For more information on knitting for charity, visit www.woolworks.org/charity.html. Vicki teaches middle school gifted students and lives with her husband and two boys. Visit her Web site at www.applesandchalkdust.com.

Prayers on Rest

Lord, make me a channel of your peace.
Where there is hatred, let me bring love.
Where there is offense, forgiveness.
Where there is discord, reconciliation.
Where there is doubt, faith.
Where there is sadness, joy.
Where there is darkness, your light.
If we give, we are made rich.
If we forget ourselves, we find peace.
If we forgive, we receive forgiveness.
If we die, we receive eternal resurrection.
Give us peace, Lord.[9]

———

God, give me the serenity to accept things
which cannot be changed;
Give me courage to change things
which must be changed;
And the wisdom to distinguish one from the other.[10]

———

I asked God for strength, that I might achieve
I was made weak, that I might learn humbly to obey . . .

I asked for health, that I might do greater things
I was given infirmity, that I might do better things . . .
I asked for riches, that I might be happy
I was given poverty, that I might be wise . . .
I asked for power, that I might have the praise of men
I was given weakness, that I might feel the need of God . . .
I asked for all things, that I might enjoy life
I was given life, that I might enjoy all things . . .
I got nothing that I asked for—but everything I had hoped for.
Almost despite myself, my unspoken prayers were answered.
I am, among all men, most richly blessed.[11]

———

The LORD is my shepherd; there is nothing I lack.
He lets me lie down in green pastures;
He leads me beside quiet waters.
He renews my life;
He leads me along the right paths
for His name's sake.
Even when I go
through the darkest valley,
I fear no danger,
for You are with me;
Your rod and Your staff—
they comfort me.
PSALM 23:1–4

———

God, create a clean heart for me
and renew a steadfast spirit within me.

Do not banish me from Your presence
or take Your Holy Spirit from me.
Restore the joy of Your salvation to me,
and give me a willing spirit.
PSALM 51:10–12

Resources for Rest

Ecclesiastes: A Time for Everything:
  7 Studies for Individuals or Groups
By Stephen Board
A Fisherman Bible Studyguide
WaterBrook Press (Colorado Springs, Colo.), 2000

Rest Stops for Teachers
By Susan Titus Osborn
Broadman & Holman Publishers (Nashville, Tenn.), 2003

Celebrating the Sabbath: Finding Rest in a Restless World
By Bruce A. Ray
P&R Publishing (Phillipsburg, N.J.), 2000

When Women Long for Rest
By Cindi McMenamin
Harvest House Publishers (Eugene, Ore.), 2004

Daily PrayerWalk: Meditations for a Deeper Prayer Life
By Janet Holm McHenry
WaterBrook Press (Colorado Springs, Colo.), 2002

A Quiet Place in a Crazy World
By Joni Eareckson Tada
Multnomah Publishers (Sisters, Ore.), 1993

He Leads Me Beside Still Waters:
    A Forty-Day Journey toward Rest for Your Soul
By Jennifer Kennedy Dean
Broadman & Holman Publishers (Nashville, Tenn.), 2001

Lord, I'm Torn between Two Masters
By Kay Arthur
Multnomah Publishers (Sisters, Ore.), 1996

5-Minute Retreats for Women
By Sue Augustine
Harvest House Publishers (Eugene, Ore.), 2001

Busy but Balanced
By Mimi Doe
St. Martin's Press (New York), 2001

Living Well with Chronic Fatigue Syndrome and Fibromyalgia
By Mary J. Shomon
HarperCollins Publishers (New York), 2004

Schools with Spirit:
    Nurturing the Inner Lives of Children and Teachers
Linda Lantieri, editor
Beacon Press (Boston), 2001

Restless Till We Rest in You
St. Augustine
Servant Publications (Ann Arbor, Mich.), 1998

Beating Busyness
By Adam R. Holz
NavPress (Colorado Springs, Colo.), 1999

The Contemplative Mom: Restoring Rich Relationship
    with God in the Midst of Motherhood
By Ann Kroeker
WaterBrook Press (Colorado Springs, Colo.), 2000

The Simple Living Guide
By Janet Luhrs
Broadway Books (New York), 1997

Energy Plan
By Aliza Baron Cohen
Laurel Glen (San Diego, Calif.), 2002

Tired of Being Tired: Rescue, Repair, Rejuvenate
By Jesse Lynn Hanley, M.D., and Nancy DeVille
G.P. Putnam's Sons (New York), 2001

Notes

1. Center for the Voice: Professions at Risk (New York Eye and Ear Infirmary), www.nyee.edu/cfv-professions.html.

2. Jesse Lynn Hanley, M.D., and Nancy DeVille, *Tired of Being Tired* (New York: Putnam, 2001).

3. Robert J. Marzano, *A Different Kind of Classroom* (Alexandria, Va.: Association for Supervision and Curriculum Development, 1992).

4. Hanley and DeVille, *Tired,* 179.

5. Richard Schramm, "How Do We Retain Our Teachers?" *Raleigh (N.C.) News,* October 13, 1995.

6. *Gotham Gazette,* April 4, 2003, www.gothamgazette .com/article/20030407/202/339.

7. "Stress forces teachers to quit," BBC News online, http://news.bbc.co.uk/1/low/education/660906.stm, February 29, 2000.

8. Karen Lurie, "Keeping Teachers," *ScienCentralNews,* May 27, 2004.

9. Prayer of St. Francis (of Assisi), Auspicious van Corstanje, *Francis: Bible of the Poor* (Chicago: Franciscan Herald Press, 1977), 203.

10. Reinhold Niebuhr, "The Serenity Prayer," *The AA Grapevine,* January 1950, 6–7; www.aagrapevine.org.

11. Author unknown. As "A Creed for Those Who Have Suffered," this has been used by rehabilitation centers. Adlai E. Stevenson used these lines on his Christmas card, 1955.